THE SUPER 500
RAPID WEIGHT LOSS
PROGRAM

THE SUPER 500 RAPID WEIGHT LOSS PROGRAM

Ronald R. Romano, D.C.

PARKER PUBLISHING COMPANY, INC.
West Nyack, NY

Library of Congress Cataloging in Publication Data

Romano, Ronald R
  The super 500 rapid weight loss program.

Includes index.
  1. Reducing diets. 2. Nutrition. I. Title.
RM222.2.R64   613.2'5   80-29466
ISBN 0-13-875930-8

Printed in the United States of America

Dedicated to
Nanny & Poppy

A WORD FROM THE AUTHOR

The following pages contain all the information you will ever need to lose weight and maintain slenderness. I have worked diligently, over a period of many months, to include every pertinent detail regarding the Super 500 Rapid Weight Loss Program.

As you read through these pages, I am sure you will be excited and pleased to learn about the experiences of many of my patients. These patients are not unlike yourself. Some of them needed to lose only a few pounds while others required weight losses in excess of fifty pounds. Yet in each instance, these patients faced the same problems and experienced the same anxiety you are presently feeling.

Please don't be concerned or anxious. Be assured that once you have finished reading this book, once you have implemented the Super 500 Rapid Weight Loss Program, you too will quickly achieve your desired weight.

When you read how Sharon forced me to include sweet and delicious thickshakes into her program, or how Diane C. continued her "eating out" life style and still lost 27 pounds, you will be able to identify with these once-overweight individuals.

The problems and disappointments which face the average overweight person are almost universal, and I am sure you will be able to empathize with most (if not all) of the experiences I relate in the following pages. At the same time, I know you will laugh and rejoice once you learn the means by which these problems and disappointments are eradicated. As you read about Jim K., and suddenly realize that

7

his craving for chocolate donuts is not unlike your own desire for certain foods, you will immediately identify with him and the problem he faced. You will, by being exposed to his solution, quickly formulate your own, and be heartened by the fabulous results achieved.

Never allow yourself to think you are alone. Remember that although you are a unique and important human being, your concerns about obesity and dieting are shared by thousands. Remember also that the Super 500 Program will quickly reverse your obese condition, and that in a very short time you will wonder why you ever allowed yourself to become overweight.

Now, before you get into the body of the book, I would like to bring together for you all the essential parts of the Super 500 Rapid Weight Loss Program. Although each of these points is covered in greater detail in the following pages, it will benefit you to have a basic understanding of how and why the Super 500 Program is so successful in reducing weight.

Basically, the only thing you really need know is why I have named this reducing procedure the Super 500 Rapid Weight Loss Program.

First of all, I use the term *Super* because this program allows you to eat approximately 875 calories per day, while permitting the utilization of only about 375 of those calories. To me, this *is* SUPER. This apparent enigma is primarily the result of what is called the Specific Dynamic Action (SDA) of foods, and since the biochemical and physiological aspects of this process is quite elaborate and complex, I will forego a detailed description of it. For those who are truly interested in precisely how it works I refer you to any standard physiology text.

Additionally, I have included the number 500 in the title for three very important reasons. First, because the entire program lasts only 500 hours (less than three weeks); second, because each day you will be eating a minimum of 500 grams of carbohydrate foods (ie., starches, sugars); and third, because you will also be consuming at least 500 calories of protein foods (ie., meat, fish, etc.).

Finally, I include the term Rapid because any dietary program that only takes three weeks to produce dramatic and noticeable results *is* rapid.

If you keep these facts in mind as you begin your weight reduction, you will have no problem following this exciting program to its successful conclusion.

In closing, let me suggest that you take a photograph of yourself today (for memory's sake), for in three weeks you will hardly recognize your slender new body.

Dr. Ronald R. Romano

CONTENTS

CHAPTER 1

HOW THE SUPER 500 PROGRAM PREVENTS FAILURE

To me there is nothing more exciting or stimulating to an obese person than the contemplation of slenderness. Nothing seizes the imagination or offers greater rewards than that single word—**SLENDERNESS**. If you are anything like the majority of my patients, you have undoubtedly faced months, or perhaps even years of fighting the "battle of the bulge." You have attempted to lose weight, and probably have been partially successful. Unfortunately, however, you have regained all those extra pounds you once lost, and although you are again contemplating the pleasures of slenderness, you dread the austerity of dieting.

Take heart! Slenderness, with all its attendant rewards, can now be yours, and yours for life. You will never again be bothered by unsightly bulges, flabby thighs, or a pendulous abdomen. You will be able to take pride in your appearance, become active (without being self-conscious), and enjoy meeting new people. In effect, you will once again become an enthusiastic participant in the game of life.

I realize that you have probably heard all of this before, and you are probably skeptical. I know that you have been disappointed in the past, and therefore read these words with a degree of cynicism. Let me assure you though, that the *Super 500 Rapid Weight Loss Program* is like nothing you've ever seen before. You will be amazed at the ease with which you lose weight. As the pounds virtually melt from your body, you will experience a revitalization; a resurgence of energy. You will be astonished at how quickly your body takes on the svelte appearance of youth. As those around you comment on your new-found slenderness, you will begin to acknowledge and accept yourself for the valuable person you are.

I know that now, even at this very moment, you probably fantasize about how your life would change, if only you could lose those excess pounds. With the Super 500 Program at your disposal, those fantasies no longer need be relegated to daydreams. Your slender new body awaits you; it is just around the corner. In three weeks or less, you can lose as many as 50 pounds. Imagine what the loss of that much weight would do for *your* figure. Imagine how differently you would feel about yourself. Imagine, if you will (and just for a moment), the inner excitement you would experience should your long-held fantasies become reality in less than a month.

Not only is all this possible: it is virtually guaranteed. If you will but read and use the information contained in the following pages, you will attain your slenderness goal in short order. You will never again be embarrassed by your obesity, nor will you avoid contact with others because you are ashamed of your shape. A new life awaits you!

Why Rapid Reduction Is Important

Although it has perhaps taken you years to attain your present weight, you would be the rare individual indeed if you did not want to lose all your excess pounds as rapidly as possible. Diet programs that promise *gradual* weight loss are rarely successful. Let's face it! Right now you are discontented with your appearance, and if that appearance is not quickly altered by your efforts to follow a dietary regimen, you will cast the regimen aside and search for a better, more rapid weight-loss program. No one can blame you for your seemingly impatient attitude. *Now* is when you are unhappy with your appearance, and *now* is when you want to change it. That is why rapid weight reduction is so important.

Given your "druthers," I believe you'd "druther" be slender right now, instead of having to wait a year, or maybe even two. How much more exciting life would be if you could look forward to a new, slender physique in just a few weeks. Think of the pleasure you'd experience if an aquaintance you hadn't seen for a month or so failed to recognize you. Nothing could be more satisfying! This one factor—the speed with which you shed those excess pounds—is extremely important.

To bring this point home, I would like to relate the story of Pam L. Since this happened just recently, I am changing the story slightly so as not to embarrass anyone.

Pam, who had been a patient of mine for some time, finally decided to lose weight. She had been obese for most of her adult life, and now, at the age of 42, felt compelled to do something about her figure. Pam was more than 47 pounds overweight, and although her 5'6" frame did help her to carry that excess weight quite nicely, she was decidedly obese. Once she decided to do something about her figure however, Pam forged right ahead. In slightly over a month, Pam reduced her weight so dramatically (42 pounds), that at a meeting of the Women's Auxiliary to a local hospital, she was asked to leave.

It seems that at each meeting of the Auxiliary, a member of the clergy is invited to offer Benediction. Since Pam was secretary for the Auxiliary, she sat on the dais, and on this particular occasion, took her usual seat. She turned and started chatting with Reverend "Smith" seated next to her, who she had met a few times over the previous several years. Unfortunately, Reverend "Smith," who I am sure should have his eyeglass prescription checked, became quite disturbed by this annoying stranger who apparently knew quite a bit about his personal life. In short order, the good reverend turned away from Pam, and tried to ignore her.

Pam however, didn't have the faintest notion that the reverend was upset. She continued to talk, asking questions about the reverend's wife, family, etc., until finally, in exasperation, the reverend turned to Pam, and in no uncertain terms said: "Mind your own business." Pam was flabbergasted! Before she could respond to the reverend's uncalled for rudeness, he requested that she either change her seat or leave the meeting.

Pam started to chuckle. As she began to realize that the reverend didn't recognize her, she just couldn't help herself; she burst into full laughter. Unfortunately, the reverend didn't see the humor in the situation and *demanded* that Pam change her seat.

It took several minutes for Pam to calm the reverend down and explain her "mistaken identity." Once she had done so, however, the reverend turned purple with embarrassment, and apologized profusely. Finally, after trying to clear himself of any blame in not recognizing Pam, he scolded her for not telling him that she was going to lose weight.

Perhaps you will never experience the happiness Pam felt when she finally realized the reverend didn't recognize her because of her new-found slenderness, but I am sure that, once you achieve your ideal weight, similar experiences will transpire and you will feel a certain exhilaration at not being readily recognized by certain acquaintances.

The rapidity with which you lose that excess weight will be responsible for just such occurrences.

How Having Your Hunger Satisfied Makes Weight Loss Easy

Nothing, except perhaps having wet, cold feet, is more aggravating than prolonged hunger. The gnawing, growling stomach that is associated with most diets does more to cause the failure of diet programs than any other single factor. Fortunately, from Day One on the *Super 500 Rapid Weight Loss Program*, you will never feel this discomfort.

Be honest: isn't one of the reasons you've given up on other diets the fact that you were constantly hungry? In my experience, the repeated, unsatisfied cravings for certain foods (or even just adequate food), has caused more people to give up on their diets than any other factor. There is good reason for this!

Most overweight individuals have enormous amounts of perseverance. They could easily follow any dietary regimen for a specified period of time, so long as they could see the light at the end of the tunnel. Unless dieters can be assured that they will soon be able to return to a normal life style, and all that it represents, there is just no way to reinforce their motivation. At the same time, if a diet represents major sacrifices in the quantity and quality of food that is permitted, and to dieters this sacrifice will have to be made for the rest of their lives, failure is almost guaranteed. No one is willing to sacrifice the enjoyment of good food and drink for *LIFE*. At least I haven't met them as yet.

This is where the Super 500 Program really excels. From the very first day on the program, you will eat as much, if not more, than you already eat. Not only will you be eating more: you will also be eating *good* food that is delicious and nutritious. I honestly don't think you could ask for a better program. To enjoy three full meals each day, to be able to eat three satisfying snacks without having to exercise, and still lose weight faster than you ever dreamed possible, is just "too good to be true." But it is true, as you will soon find out.

Over the past fourteen years, I have successfully treated numerous overweight patients; but until the advent of the *Super 500 Rapid Weight Loss Program*, not one of them ever told me they truly enjoyed themselves while dieting, and were going to continue with my recommendations indefinitely. What more "testimony" could any dietary program have, than that the dieters want to remain on it even after they've achieved their proper weight?

How Results Really Motivate

The measure of any program is its results. When talking about diets, the results are measured in pounds and inches. Nothing else matters. It makes no difference that a diet is easy or pleasurable; it remains a failure if you do not lose the desired amount of weight. In reality, for any dietary program to be successful, it must culminate in slenderness.

How many times in the past have you tried to lose weight and failed because you were dissatisfied with the results achieved? I don't blame you! Only masochists would want to deny themselves the pleasure of food and drink without the reward of becoming slender. Sometimes, even when results are evident, they are often insufficient to warrant continuation on the particular diet. To diet for a month or more, to notice only a weight loss of 8 or 10 pounds, is horrifying. Only rapid and substantial weight loss will re-motivate you to diet for the next day or week. Since the Super 500 Program produces almost immediate results—immediate loss of pounds and inches—you will have no problem remaining on the program. Each day, as your scale registers lower and lower weight, you will be repeatedly stimulated to continue on to your ultimate goal: **slenderness.** As your clothing begins to hang on you, when you have difficulty holding up your pants, you will need little more to "psych" yourself into continuing with the program. Nothing is more capable of keeping you on a diet than the loss of those unwanted pounds. In less than three weeks, you will understand what I am saying better than if I spent three hours trying to explain it. **Slenderness is its own reward!**

Solving the Obesity Problem

Every doctor is continually bombarded by patients requesting help with their weight problems. Unfortunately, most doctors ignore their patients' pleas in this regard, or, at the very most, offer some vague, pre-printed dietary format as the solution to obesity. If you have consulted your own physician in the past, you can probably back me up on this. It seems that, although every doctor will readily admit obesity presents a major health problem, few will take the time or have the interest to actively assist their patients in losing weight. I, for one, am at a loss to explain this enigma. Patients suffering from continued obesity require as much, if not more, help to overcome their condition, as patients with "essential" gastroenteritis. To offer only a kind word, a pat on the back, and a pre-printed form that promises the loss of a pound or two per week, is inadequate. The obese patient needs more, much more!

During the past fourteen years of practice, I have often been asked if there was something *new* that could help the overweight individual. This book answers that question, and the answer is **yes!** There is something new; it's called the *Super 500 Rapid Weight Loss Program*, and it makes all other dietary programs seem worthless by comparison.

The Super 500 Program didn't come into being by some ingenious stroke of luck, nor did it present itself to me in the form of a complete, effective approach to the problem of obesity. Instead, the program came about through the efforts of patients much like yourself. These patients and their desire for slenderness, led to the formulation of the Super 500 Program.

Only a totally insensitive person can repeatedly ignore the requests of others, and since I consider myself a dedicated and caring physician, it didn't take long for me to become completely involved in trying to find a solution to the problem of obesity. As the program evolved, patient "feedback" became increasingly important. At times, it seemed that every step forward resulted in two steps backward. Without the continued support of patients, without their suggestions, the *Super 500 Rapid Weight Loss Program* would never have seen the light of day. The number of formerly obese patients who helped perfect the Super 500 Program is too great for me to thank each one individually. Each of you knows who you are, and how much I appreciate your assistance.

How the Super 500 Program
Overcomes Major Stumbling Blocks

When I first began my investigation into methods of controlling obesity, I was completely unaware of the magnitude of the problems I would encounter. Initially, my recommendations to patients consisted primarily of calorie-restricted diets. It didn't take long, however, for me to discover the inadequacy of such approaches. Each returning patient reported new and different problems with the diets I had prescribed. At first I thought these problems would disappear by themselves, but I soon recognized the foolishness of this belief. Once I realized that the problems my patients were reporting were real, I took steps to eliminate them.

I began to classify objections to the diets in a standardized manner. I analyzed and re-analyzed the terminology that patients used to describe their discontent. Once I had received a minimum of three objections to any particular aspect of a diet, I took immediate steps to remove that "rule" from the program. As the months went by, I found that my original program had evolved to a point where it was no longer recognizable. In less than a year, I had produced a dietary program unlike any other. By using a multiple-technique approach to weight reduction, I had synthesized a regimen that:

1) Takes only 500 hours to produce dramatic weight loss (approximately twenty-one days).
2) Effectively eliminates any feeling of hunger.
3) Permits the dieter to eat snacks, "junk-food," etc.
4) Is safe for everyone—even those individuals who have physical disorders.
5) Does not require any exercise to be effective.
6) Allows the dieter to eat out at restaurants, fast-food establishments, etc.
7) Eliminates "Dieter's Depression."
8) Allows spot-reducing to take place automatically.

Once this dietary regimen became fully operational, patient after obese patient reported amazing results. The pounds and inches melted from their bodies as never before. Enthusiasm reigned supreme!

If you wish to lose those unsightly pounds faster than you dreamed possible, if you want to feel energetic and excited about dieting, if you want to do all this without exercise, the *Super 500 Rapid Weight Loss Program* is for you. It works better than anything else available. I'm sure you will be pleased with the results it will achieve for you.

CHAPTER 2

THE DYNAMICS OF
THE SUPER 500
RAPID WEIGHT LOSS PROGRAM

I am sure that you want to obtain maximum results with the Super 500 Program, and unless I am mistaken, you would like to lose all your excess weight as quickly as possible. You wish to become slender and proud of your shape. To do this, you must first understand the basic premise upon which the Super 500 Program is based. Without that understanding, you will undoubtedly prolong your reducing program, and perhaps even regain the pounds you've lost once you are on your own, eating the foods you like.

Please don't be apprehensive about the need to understand how the Super 500 works. You will find that by reading the following material, you will have a totally effective, working knowledge of the rationale behind the Super 500. Although this program is based on complex biochemical and neurophysiological concepts, there is no need to burden you with a step-by-step description of these processes. As long as you understand the *do's* and *don'ts* of the program, you will have no trouble losing all the weight you want. As I said before, your new slender body awaits you; it is only three weeks away.

Why Certain Foods Are Essential

All living organisms require certain specific conditions if life is to be maintained. For the human body, air (oxygen) and water are essential. Without oxygen, human life would end in just a few minutes. Water, although not as necessary as oxygen from a time standpoint, is no less important to life. If you were denied access to water, you would only be able to function for several days, after which life would cease. Although air and water are primary, the human body also requires other factors for its continuation. Among these are vitamins, minerals, essential fatty acids and amino acids. In order to live a full and healthy life, the foods you eat must supply these factors. Without them, you will produce definite, pre-determined bodily dysfunction. To prevent this from ever occurring, certain foods (as well as other factors) must be included in any dietary program you attempt.

Perhaps the most important factors relative to continued good health are vitamins and minerals. I am sure you have heard much about these; you are probably even tired of hearing about them. Without trying your patience, let me explain that you *must* take a vitamin/mineral supplement while on the Super 500 Program. I won't go into a long explanation of the whys and wherefores; just be assured that this recommendation must be followed if you wish to lose weight *rapidly*. In a following chapter, I will explain exactly which vitamin/mineral supplement to take, and how to take it.

The second and third factors to be considered are the essential fatty acids and amino acids. These have been generally overlooked by individuals who promulgate "fad" diets, but they are just as necessary as vitamins and minerals. Once again, I will not bore you with all the details: just be assured that these factors are necessary to good health and have been included in the proper amounts within the *Super 500 Rapid Weight Loss Program.*

Why Ken R. Found the Super 500 Beautiful

Ken is probably one of the most enthusiastic supporters of the Super 500. For years he had unsuccessfully tried to lose thirty pounds, located mainly in his abdomen. Ken had the typical "beer belly." Every time he tried to lose weight, he found himself exhausted, and since he worked as a concrete-laborer foreman, Ken needed all the strength and energy he could muster. Yet, because diets had always caused him to feel weak and tired by the middle of the first afternoon on any diet, Ken lost all motivation and began to eat and drink as before. Time and time again, Ken resolved to do better and get rid of his "beer belly."

Unfortunately, the harder he tried to lose those excess pounds, the more firmly they seemed to be attached to him. Ken had almost lost all his desire to lose weight when another patient of mine told him about the Super 500 and how it had helped her lose 27 pounds.

On his first visit to my office, Ken told me of his previous attempts at weight loss. He explained the difficulties he had encountered, as well as his dieting experiences. It seems that every time Ken tried to lose weight, he would get dizzy spells which usually would start a few hours after breakfast. First he would notice light-headedness, which quickly became a full-blown dizzy spell. Ken always feared that he would "black out" during one of these periods, and since his work involved heavy construction equipment, he was afraid that he could be injured. I quickly put Ken's mind at ease, explaining that during the Super 500 Program, he would not experience any untoward effects. The reason he had previously been bothered by dizziness was low blood sugar. Since the Super 500 Program takes this problem into account and precludes its ever occurring, Ken would have no problem.

After examining him and determining that there was no reason why Ken couldn't lose his excess weight, I explained the Super 500 Program. While doing this, I described one of the satisfiers (ie., Creamy Banana Thick Shake) that would be included in his daily food intake. Ken was astounded.

"How can I possibly lose weight when I'm allowed to eat foods like that?" he asked.

"Don't worry about it. The pounds will come off," I reassured him.

Nineteen days later, Ken returned to the office. He had lost 28 pounds and was ecstatic.

"I never would have believed it," he began. "If anyone would have told me that I could lose all that weight in so short a time, I would have laughed at him.

"I still can't believe it. During the past two and a half weeks, I've felt great; I've been eating everything on the diet, especially the satisfiers, and I still lost more than I'd expected. Those satisfiers are fabulous. Everytime I had one, I felt like a little kid stealing from the cookie jar.

"Doc, all I can say is, the Super 500 Program is beautiful."

It's nine months since Ken lost those pounds and that "beer belly," and today he looks just as super as he did on the day he returned to my office 28 pounds lighter. Every time I see Ken, he just shakes his head in disbelief and repeats, "Beautiful, just beautiful."

Although Ken thinks the Super 500 Program is a miracle, the results he achieved are not unusual. Many patients have lost 25, 30, even 40 pounds in less than three weeks, and continue to maintain their slender new figures indefinitely. I am sure that your experience with the Super 500 will be just as successful and just as exciting.

How the 500 Program Forces the Body to Burn Fat

Perhaps one of the truly amazing features of the 500 program is that it permits you to eat adequate quantities of food, without allowing you to utilize all the calories contained in the food you eat. This is accomplished through a well-recognized process known as the specific dynamic action of foods. Don't let the term throw you. There is nothing mysterious about this process. Although physiologists are still confused as to why this process occurs, they are completely in agreement about how it works.

Let me give you a simple example of how the specific

dynamic action (SDA) of protein works. Assume for the moment, that your body burns calories at the rate of ten per hour. This means that in twenty-four hours, you would burn up 240 calories. If, however, you were to consume some high-protein food, your body would start to burn thirteen calories an hour, or 312 calories per day. That's right! By eating high protein foods, you force your body to burn at least an additional 30 percent of the calories normally burned. Think about that for a moment.

What I am saying is, that if you consume protein foods equal to 30 percent of your normal daily caloric output, in effect, you will have eaten nothing at all. The food you eat is offset by the increased rate of output. You would, therefore, be in nutritional balance. Any activity (walking, work, cooking, etc.) that you perform in addition to just lying around all day, would additionally increase the amount of calories you are burning and thus result in a negative nutritional state (i.e., you would be burning more calories than you are consuming); therefore, your body would have to draw on your fat reserves to provide these additional calories. Every time you were to do this, you would actually be losing weight as your body was forced to use its own stores of fat.

Although this may seem impossible to you, it is a medical fact. Any physician, biochemist, or physiologist will be happy to back me up. You can find additional information on this unique process in any medical physiology text.

There is a "catch" though. The specific dynamic action of protein can be easily offset by taking in other foods at the same time as you eat the protein. Only a properly balanced intake of protein, fats and carbohydrates will produce the results you want. That is why the Super 500 Program is so successful. It provides for a precisely balanced intake of foods while at the same time taking advantage of this process. In addition, the Super 500 relies on the dynamic action of fats and carbohydrates, which although not as great as protein, also produce additional caloric output.

In effect then, the Super 500 Program forces you to burn up that excess fat by chemical means, not physical activity.

That is why exercise, as such, is uncalled for when losing weight on this program. Once you understand the importance of this process and the way it works, you will have no trouble taking off all those excess pounds.

Even after the program is complete and you have attained your ideal weight, you will have no trouble maintaining that weight. Just follow what you already know (and what you will soon learn) about the specific dynamic action of foods.

How Necessary Calories Are Included in the Super 500 Program

Calories are nothing more than the way scientists measure the energy content of foods. If a food provides a lot of energy, it has a high calorie content. On the other hand, if a food produces little energy, it is considered to have few calories. The unfortunate thing about calories is that most people enjoy those foods which contain the greatest number of them. For instance, pure fat contains more than twice the calories of protein or carbohydrate foods. That is why butter, mayonaise, bacon, fried foods, etc., are eliminated from most diets. These foods contain a high proportion of fat, and are therefore very high in caloric content; twice as high as other, non-fat foods.

There is no use bemoaning this fact however, since there is little we can do about it. If we are to function normally, if we are to have the energy necessary for our everyday activities, we must have calories included in our daily intake of food. The only thing we can do is balance the number of calories against our utilization of them. By this I mean that we must consume the exact (or nearly exact) number of calories we expend each day. If we can determine how much energy you normally burn, and then permit you to eat just the right amount of calories to offset that energy expenditure, we can force you to lose weight. This is because the specific dynamic action of food increases the number of calories you normally burn, without you even being aware of it.

What better approach could you ask for: the number of calories you normally burn up each day through your normal routine is being continually replenished, yet you still lose weight because of that process known as specific dynamic action.

As I said before, you must have adequate calories if you want to continue doing everything you normally do without feeling tired or irritable. But if we can supply a major portion of those necessary calories, through the use of protein foods, and thereby increase the rate at which our bodies burn up energy, we will put ourselves into negative nutritional balance and thereby reduce our weight. This fact alone is a prerequisite to successful dieting, and that is why it is included as a major part of the *Super 500 Rapid Weight Loss Program.*

Chapter 3

HOW THE SUPER 500 PROGRAM REMOVES POUNDS WITHOUT DRUDGERY

If you are anything like my overweight patients, you have probably tried, on numerous occasions, to lose weight. Perhaps you have been successful, or at least partially successful in the past. Today however, you have probably regained most, if not all, of the weight you previously lost. You are once again facing the need to diet.

If you no longer wish to restrict your food intake in order to lose weight, if you just can't get excited about the prospects of strenuous exercise in order to trim down, then the information in this book is important to you.

Every time you try to accomplish some feat, you must be adequately motivated and be capable of altering your life style so as to produce the desired results. If the task you are attempting is such that intermediate goals can be determined and measured, you should have little difficulty in maintaining adequate motivation. In any dietary program, these intermediate goals are represented by the number of pounds and inches lost from your body. Unfortunately, most programs concerned with weight reduction are overly restrictive. They do not permit much leeway in the quantity or variety of the foods allowed. This fact alone results in the diet becoming a tedious experience.

The fact that your physical activities and life style regarding food intake are regimented, produces stress that is uncalled for. Although your motivation may be maintained by the results you achieve, the boredom and drudgery of having to eat the same foods, day in and day out, often lead to failure. The *Super 500 Rapid Weight Loss Program* has been developed to provide continuous variety.

Each day of the program, each meal and snack, has been designed to offer you the greatest latitude in choosing what you wish to eat. You will find that within the broad parameters specified by the Super 500 Program, you will be able to choose physical activities, food, and drink you previously thought were inconsistent with dieting.

Why Variety Is So Important

Most dieters rarely take the time to consider the importance of variety. Most of them will complain that a particular diet is too difficult to live with. They may even indicate that it is something about the foods permitted that causes them to discard a specific dietary program. In almost every instance, however, the lack of variety in the foods permitted is the causative factor behind the dieter's reluctance to continue on the program.

When I speak of variety, I am referring not only to the flavor of food, but also to its consistency. This area is usually overlooked. Perhaps an example of what I mean will help illustrate the importance of this concept.

Imagine for a moment that you were permitted to eat any and all, fresh, leafy, green vegetables. Although each vegetable has its distinct flavor, its consistency would be almost the same as any other green, leafy vegetable. For instance, Iceberg lettuce, Bibb lettuce, Boston lettuce, kale and escarole are all green, leafy vegetables, and each has a distinct flavor. Unfortunately, they all have the same basic consistency, and if you ate them on a repetitive basis, you would soon grow tired of them. I think you can see, therefore, that not only is the flavor of the food important, but also its consistency. The *Super 500 Rapid Weight Loss Program* is designed to take this fact into consideration. While following the program, you will find that the foods included provide a great variety, not only in flavor and aroma, but also in consistency. By including these foods, I have attempted to instill a certain excitement and variety in the daily meal programs.

How to Diet Without Boredom

Many of my patients have told me that in the past, dieting was a lonely and often boring experience. They reported that while losing weight on the Super 500 Program, they were able to maintain a high degree of motivation and excitement about their weight loss. The reason for this, at least in part, was the reinforcement they received by repetitive visits to my office, by the ability to discuss problems as they came up, and the constant monitoring of their progress.

In an effort to make this program as reinforcing and interesting as the personally supervised program I use in my office, I have tried to include much of the advice that I would normally give to my patients. I have done this on a day-to-day basis, instead of trying to give you everything "up-front." In this way, as you proceed with the program and experience new and different feelings, you will have the benefit of my advice on a continuous basis. In addition, I have also included almost every question I could recall that patients have asked me regarding dieting. I have answered these in another chapter, and I recommend that if you have a particular question regarding your own experiences during the program, you turn to that section and find the answers.

The inclusion of "feedback" on a continuous basis through the daily "Notes" section of the dietary program, along with the answers to your questions as they arise, will undoubtedly provide repetitive stimulation for you. I have tried to include some interesting anecdotes and intriguing recipes within the program, since I feel that this will make your brief involvement with the Super 500 more interesting.

How Satiety Makes Weight Loss Enjoyable

In the past, every time you attempted to lose weight, you were most likely faced with the spectre of continued, prolonged hunger. Not so on the 500 Program. The 500 Program has been designed so that the foods permitted will produce satisfaction, and satiety. In this way, once you have eaten the foods permitted on the program, there will be no physical cravings for additional foods. In addition, to prevent any psychological or emotional cravings for additional food, I have included a variety of delicious snacks and desserts. These have come to be known as "Satisfiers" since most patients have reported that they truly do satisfy cravings for sweets, snacks, and "munchies" during the course of the program.

If, while you are losing weight, you notice that you do feel hungry, it is imperative that you try to discover the cause of this hunger. Since there are adequate quantities of food, and more than sufficient snacks included in the program, the most likely reason for hunger would be that you have either skipped a meal or a satisfier. I caution you to try to not do this. Missing a meal normally results in increased cravings for food at the next mealtime, and this often leads to over-indulgence. If you will eat everything permitted, you will have no trouble, and will honestly enjoy losing those excess pounds.

I have often found that the main reason individuals fail to lose weight on any dietary program is a feeling that they are denying themselves. Be assured that if you eat all the foods allowed on the Super 500, you will have no cravings for additional "forbidden" foods. Skipping individual meals will only produce greater stress, and will not necessarily accelerate the speed with which you lose weight. Enjoy yourself; the Super 500 Program has been designed to produce rapid and sustained weight loss. There is no need for you to alter or modify the program.

The Satisfier and How It Works

Although many obese individuals are not "sweets" eaters, I have found that these individuals overindulge at their regular mealtimes. For the few overweight individuals who do enjoy snacking, the cause of their obesity is usually the calories contained in those snacks. It would appear, therefore, that we are faced with two distinct problems; on the one hand we have the individual who does not snack but overeats at meals, and on the other hand we have the individual who perhaps does not overeat at mealtime, but who enjoys continuous or intermittent snacking between meals. Both conditions result in a gain and maintenance of increased weight.

The satisfier is designed to help both these individuals. For the person who enjoys between-meal snacks, the satisfier will be a refreshing break from the ordinary. For those individuals who overeat at regular meal times, the satisfier acts as an appetite suppressant, thereby precluding over-indulgence at regular mealtime.

I am sure you will find the satisfiers to be both enjoyable and delicious, as well as satisfying. When eaten routinely as directed, the satisfiers will serve their intended purpose. The individual who enjoys snacking will be satisfied, and the individual who overeats at mealtime will have a lessened appetite. I recommend, therefore, that where permitted, you indulge yourself and enjoy the "Satisfiers."

Why No "Down Time" Means Fast Results

In the previous chapter, I related the story of Ken R. If you recall, Ken was bothered by light-headedness and dizziness every time he had previously tried to diet. These symptoms are not uncommon. They are caused by a lowering of the blood-sugar level between meals. The satisfiers, with their high content of carbohydrate calories, are intended to prevent this from happening. Unfortunately, there are times and instances when taking a satisfier is impossible. I have therefore included a substitute for them. By taking this substitute, you will have no problem with low blood sugar and therefore will not have dizziness, light-headedness, or the other most common symptom, depression. While losing weight on the Super 500 Program, you will have no "down time." You will not feel depressed, or denied. You will be able to maintain your energy levels and your excitement for life. It is essential, though, that you follow the recommendations of the program, and either consume the satisfiers as prescribed or substitute the Super 500 Energizer which is described in a later chapter.

Why You will Feel Better with Every Pound You Lose

Every pound of excess fat requires considerable energy to be maintained. Several miles of blood vessels and an adequate blood supply are necessary to keep those fat deposits available for use by the body. Each time you lose a pound of fat, you reduce the stress on both your heart and on your physiological homeostasis (balance) by an enormous amount. In this way, each pound of fat that is melted from your body makes available the energy normally consumed in maintaining that fat. Because of this, you will feel both energetic and strengthened with each pound that you lose. As you attain your ideal weight, you will feel better than you have ever felt before. You will attempt and accomplish new projects; projects which you have been putting off for a long time. You will find that your capacity for physical activity has greatly increased, and because of this increased energy expenditure, you will find that maintaining your new lowered weight is quite easy.

Why Theresa Tried Tennis

When Theresa first consulted me for her overweight condition, she was, in a word, "dumpy." She was only 5'4" tall, and weighed 153 pounds. She needed to lose 25 pounds in order to achieve her ideal weight. Unfortunately, Theresa had never before involved herself in physical activities: she didn't feel comfortable or graceful. Theresa was embarrassed by her obesity.

During the second week of the program, Theresa had lost 17 pounds; she felt energetic, and was no longer overly embarrassed by her excess weight. At that point, I suggested that she involve herself in some physical activity. After thinking for a few minutes, Theresa told me she had decided that she would attempt to play tennis. I reassured her that she would probably enjoy the game.

Over the next two and a half weeks, Theresa quickly lost the remaining 8 pounds of her obesity and was discharged from the office.

It was almost a year and a half before I saw Theresa once again. She had stopped by the office to say "Hi," and she looked beautiful. Her flesh was firm and her skin tanned. Her hair was partially bleached by the sun, and when she came in, she was wearing an extremely attractive tennis outfit. After a few minutes of small talk, I realized why Theresa had stopped in. She had won her first tennis tournament that morning. She minimized her achievement by praising her partner's ability, but I could see that she was extremely pleased with herself. At 27 years of age, Theresa had become a beautiful, well-proportioned woman. Her whole personality had changed: she had become outgoing, friendly, and vivacious. Losing 25 pounds had changed Theresa's whole outlook on life.

As you lose your excess weight, I know that your energy levels will increase, and that you will gain new confidence in your own ability to accomplish things and be involved with life. Perhaps you too will experience the inner satisfaction that comes from doing something well; perhaps you too will experience the pleasure of being proficient in some sport. In any event, I know you will take pride in your appearance and have a new-found excitement for living.

CHAPTER 4

THIS IS THE SUPER 500 PROGRAM

In this Chapter, I will describe the *Super 500 Rapid Weight Loss Program.* Since you are already acquainted with most of the terms and concepts from reading the previous chapters, I will try to be as concise as possible. The purpose of this chapter is to give you an overview of the complete *Super 500 Weight Loss Program.*

Read the following material carefully; it contains all the instructions necessary to initiate and follow through with rapid weight reduction. Once you've completed this chapter, you'll already be on your way to losing those excess pounds which have been annoying you; you'll be on your way to slenderness. Therefore, please take the extra few minutes necessary to read this chapter in its entirety. You will find that by doing so, you will greatly enhance your understanding of the *Super 500 Program*, and will make your rapid weight reduction both easy and enjoyable.

How Nutritional Balance Increases Weight Loss

Obesity and malnutrition seem to go hand-in-hand. Although many studies have confirmed this fact, most obese individuals still seem to believe that they eat nutritionally balanced meals. If you've been overweight since childhood, or even if your obesity is of a more recent nature, you're probably aware of and believe the general misconception that being overweight indicates proper nutritional status. This couldn't be further from the truth.

Because most overweight people pay an inordinate amount of attention to their dietary intake and consume large quantities of various foods, you would think they'd have nutritional balance. Unfortunately, most overweight individuals consume foods that do not provide the required nutritional components.

Often I have had overweight patients who literally refused to take a vitamin supplement because, they said, "Vitamins make me hungry. It's foolish to take pills that are going to make me hungry when I'm trying to lose weight."

These patients were right. The vitamins did make them hungry. This is a common effect, but it only occurs in those individuals who are *malnourished*. Don't confuse the term malnourished with undernourished: they are not the same. Malnourishment or malnutrition means bad nutrition; undernourishment or undernutrition indicates an inadequate quantity of various, required, nutritional factors. The obese individual usually is *not undernourished*, since his overweight is evidence that he's obtaining adequate quantities of food. These individuals do, however, suffer from malnutrition as a result of eating improperly. They eat foods which do not contain adequate amounts of the various required vitamins and minerals. They're definitely getting sufficient calories, but their bodies are depleted of essential vitamin constituents as evidenced by their increased hunger when taking supplements.

Although this book is not primarily concerned with physical health and disease, it is essential that you maintain a proper nutritional balance whenever you are losing weight. Since all weight reduction depends on an individual's ability to burn up more calories than he or she consumes, you can immediately recognize the need for the body to burn calories at a proper rate. Unfortunately, whenever a condition of malnutrition exists, the metabolic rate is decreased. This is a scientific fact!

Therefore, if you are suffering from a vitamin deficiency, the rate at which your body burns calories has been decreased. Thus it is easy to see why a slender person, who has a proper nutritional balance, burns up more calories than an obese person who is malnourished. Even if these two individuals were to take in an equal, predetermined amount of calories on a day-to-day basis, the obese individual would not lose weight; at the same time, the slender individual would not gain weight. This is because the slender person is burning up the excess calories quickly, while the obese individual, although his caloric intake may appear to be insufficient to maintain his obesity, burns his food at a slower pace and thus does not decrease his fat stores.

Therefore, although the *Super 500 Rapid Weight Loss Program* meets the nutritional needs of an individual, it is not sufficient to correct any underlying nutritional imbalance. Since you want to lose weight as rapidly as possible, it is important that you eliminate any malnutrition which currently exists. This is especially true while you are on the Super 500 Program.

In order to increase the rate at which you burn calories (increase your metabolic rate), vitamin supplementation is essential. This is true whether or not vitamins increase your appetite; in fact, it is especially true if you've found that vitamins increase your desire for food.

The Importance of Proper Supplementation

You are probably aware that there is an ongoing conflict between proponents of natural, organic vitamins and those who recommend synthetic products. In truth, there is no difference between the vitamins and minerals obtained from a natural organic compound and those obtained from synthetic processes. Anyone who feels that there is a difference between natural and synthetic products is unaware of the facts. Their contents are identical as stated on their labels.

There is a potential benefit, however, in taking a natural compound. A perfect illustration of this is in the case of Vitamin C. Not too many years ago, there was a conflict between proponents of natural Vitamin C and those who believed that Vitamin C obtained from a synthetic product was essentially the same. At that time, it was not known that synthetic Vitamin C was not absorbed and utilized as rapidly or as extensively as that coming from the natural product. However, it wasn't too many years later that discoveries proved that natural Vitamin C, taken from rose hips or other natural sources, contained an additional element not found in the synthetic product. This was later identified as citrus bioflavonoids. It was further demonstrated that for Vitamin C to be properly utilized, citrus bioflavonoids should be present.

This simple illustration of why a natural product is better than a synthetic (i.e., because it may contain as yet unidentified nutritional compounds that are essential to good health), should be sufficient justification for choosing a natural organic product over a synthetic one.

At this point, I feel I have adequately stressed the importance of taking vitamins, and choosing a natural organic compound as opposed to a synthetic one. All that remains is for you to purchase a product that is nutritionally complete and adequate to your needs.

You can obtain such a product at any health food store, and in most pharmacies. It may be simpler if you do not try to read and understand the entire label of each of the various products, but instead ask the pharmacist or attendant for the following:

"A complete vitamin/mineral formula, packaged in maintenance dosage."

Be sure that the word "therapeutic" is not printed anywhere on the package. What you are interested in is obtaining a product that is formulated to provide a "maintenance" dosage of the various vitamins and minerals in each tablet or capsule. Those products designed to provide therapeutic dosages are much too strong, and cannot be adequately assimilated. The high concentration of vitamins and minerals found in a therapeutic product is often irritating to the gastrointestinal tract. Thus it is better to obtain a maintenance product and take it three times a day (with food), to increase your dosage to therapeutic levels, while at the same time giving your body the opportunity to digest, absorb, and utilize the nutritional components adequately.

Therefore, on the first day of your Rapid Weight Loss Program, you will already have in your possession, a maintenance dosage vitamin/mineral formula. Throughout the program, you should take one of these vitamin/mineral tablets or capsules with each of the three "primarily protein" meals that you will be eating. I repeat: one (1) capsule or tablet with *each* "primarily protein" meal you consume.

How Pre-Programmed Meals Make Weight Loss Easy

If you are going to lose weight rapidly, your intake of food must be properly controlled. In addition, the foods in the different categories must be eaten at specific times in order to produce the desired results. To preclude any possibility of your eating more food than is required or eating the wrong foods in improper combinations, I have put together a number of meals that are nutritionally balanced, calorie controlled, and which include the proper combination of the various foods. The Super 500 Program is primarily successful in producing *rapid* weight reduction because the various food categories are consumed in a prescribed manner.

If you eat the foods that are recommended in the following program but not in the manner recommended, you will probably still lose some weight. Unfortunately, you won't lose it as rapidly, or in the enormous amounts as on the Super 500 Program. It is therefore of the utmost importance that you eat the pre-programmed meals, not only in the quantities permitted, but also in the manner prescribed. By doing this, you will find that the Super 500 Rapid Weight Loss Program is enjoyable, satisfying, and extremely quick in getting you to your slenderness goal.

In the event you wish to formulate your own meals (which I don't suggest), I have included instructions and food category lists at the end of Chapter 8. By referring to these instructions and following them *to the letter*, it is possible for you to formulate your own meals. However, I strongly recommend that, at the beginning, you utilize the pre-programmed meals as outlined. This will completely eliminate any possibility of your consuming either improper amounts or combinations of the various foods.

Understanding the Satisfier

As explained in a previous chapter, the satisfier is taken three times a day; between breakfast and lunch, between lunch and dinner, and prior to bedtime. The satisfier is primarily composed of carbohydrates. There is little or no fat or protein present in the various satisfier formulas, and there are several reasons for this.

First, a primarily carbohydrate food substantially increases energy levels. For this reason, it is recommended that the satisfier be taken at those times when energy reserves are usually low. In some instances, as you will see from the following history, another approach may be used. But in the vast majority of cases, it is recommended that you use the satisfier as outlined.

Another benefit of the satisfiers as formulated, is that they contain only minimal amounts of calories. Because of this, they can be taken in rather large quantities without inhibiting the speed of weight reduction. These quantities are satisfying both psychologically and physically, and therefore assist you in controlling your intake of food. At the same time, since there are little or no fats or proteins available in the satisfiers, the carbohydrate contents can be quickly digested, absorbed and utilized for energy conversion. This precludes the possibility of taking in excessive amounts of calories, some of which, had they been combined with protein or fat, would have been converted into fat globules for storage.

By the same token, the "primarily protein" meals you will be eating are precisely regulated. Since there will be little or no carbohydrates available at the time of eating these meals, the absorbable caloric content is minimal considering the kinds of food you'll be eating. This lack of carbohydrates at mealtime permits the Specific Dynamic Action of protein to be realized more quickly than if carbohydrates were consumed at the same time. Since the protein meals are filling and are more rapidly assimilated in the absence of carbohydrates, they will reduce your craving for food between meals.

This is both beneficial and desirable, since a reduced appetite for food between meals will permit you to take smaller quantities of the satisfiers. In this way, by taking the prescribed pre-programmed meals and satisfiers as outlined, you will be able to maintain normal energy levels while at the same time reducing caloric intake.

Because of their ability to fill, the "primarily protein" meals will prevent you from overindulging in the satisfiers; at the same time, the satisfiers will maintain your energy level and preclude your overeating at mealtime. This then is the essence of the Super 500 Rapid Weight Loss Program:

> To use specified foods which, because of their nutritional constituents, combat and counteract your need for excessive consumption of high-calorie foods, and at the same time produce an inefficiency in the way your body utilizes the foods consumed.

How Jessie L. Lost 29 Pounds By Flip-Flopping

Jessie L. was, in a word, *fat*. Her short stature made her appear heavier than she really was, and in any event, she required a weight loss of 29 pounds in order to reach her ideal weight.

When I first saw Jessie, she told me that she had attempted many, many diets, but had always been unsuccessful; they never seemed to meet her expectations.

After our initial work-up and consultations, it was decided that Jessie would do well on the Super 500 Rapid Weight Loss Program. The program was therefore outlined, and Jessie was sent on her way to lose her weight.

The following afternoon she called the Center and requested another visit. When she arrived, she told me that this "diet" was no different from any other, and that she

knew she was not going to lose any weight. After the few
minutes it took to calm her down, we discussed the benefits
of the Super 500 Program as opposed to other dietary
regimens. I soon learned that Jessie's complaint centered
around the manner in which she was to eat the "primarily
protein" meals and the satisfiers. Even with all my reas-
surances, Jessie could not see her way clear to eat a protein
meal first thing in the morning. She felt that at her age, she
couldn't change her eating habits so drastically. After several
more minutes of consultation, I learned that Jessie did feel
she could eat one of the satisfiers first thing in the morning.
As a result, I suggested that instead of having the three
"primarily protein" meals at the prescribed time, she could
change them around so that she would eat the satisfiers at
the times prescribed for the meals, and then insert the meals
into the times when she was to have her satisfiers. Jessie
agreed, and felt she could live with this. Twenty-one days
later, Jessie had lost eighteen pounds and had started on the
interim program successfully. At the end of the one-week
interim program, Jessie had lost another two pounds. She
once again reinstituted the twenty-one day Super 500 Program, and reached her ideal desirable weight two weeks
later.

The last time I saw Jessie, which was almost five months
ago, she was effusive. When I asked her what she thought of
the Super 500 Program now, Jessie answered in mock humil-
ity, "I guess it really isn't like any other diet."

I have related the story of Jessie L. to show you that
within certain limits, some of the recommendations I have
made can be altered or changed. However, the change that
was made in Jessie's regimen did not affect the basic concept
of the Super 500 Program. The meals, although switched
around, were still eaten in their proper sequence, and were
separated by an adequate period of time. If, for whatever
reason, you feel that you'd like to do the same as Jessie,
please feel free to do so. You may alter the meal and satisfier
pattern, but do not in any way alter the quantity or quality of
the food to be eaten.

How to Determine Your Ultimate Weight Loss

Over the past several years, I have had any number of overweight patients request help with their obesity. When questioned, many responded that they had to lose just a few pounds.

"How many pounds?"

"I don't know—a few. Maybe ten or twenty."

I'm bringing this up to demonstrate that it's essential for you to know exactly how many pounds you want to lose. If you wish to be successful in any venture, you must first know your ultimate goal; it's no different in weight reduction.

Before proceeding to the charts which indicate desirable weights, you should first anticipate the approximate number of pounds you wish to lose. The desirable weight charts are beneficial, but they should not be the sole determining factor in your final decision. Decide at least on a "ball park" figure before proceeding to the charts. Then, once you have decided on your ultimate weight loss goal, look at the appropriate chart.

Since you've already made a mental commitment as to your final weight goal, compare it with the indications on the chart. If you are honest with yourself, you'll probably find that there is some discrepancy between what you have already contemplated, and what the desirable weight chart states. This is almost invariably due to "setting your goals too low."

Time and time again, patients come to me and ask me to help them lose weight. When I finally discover their anticipated weight loss, there is usually a discrepancy between it and the weight charts. This is because many patients have a preconceived notion as to how they would look at a specific weight. Unfortunately, most of the time the obese person tries to pick a weight heavier than one that would be most desirable. This is because they assume it will be easier to attain their goals and to maintain that particular weight. However, this isn't true! As a matter of fact, the converse is true. If you do not achieve your ideal weight commensurate with your body proportions, you will find that you will have difficulty maintaining your weight, and will regain it much more rapidly. It's my belief that subconsciously, you will still feel fat if you do not achieve an *honest* desirable weight.

Please do not tell me that you will "look too skinny, appear drawn or sick, or look like death warmed over"; I have heard these excuses too many times. The desirable weight charts are just that, *desirable*. If you're going to lose weight, you may as well achieve the ideal instead of trying to pick a seemingly easier goal. You'll definitely like yourself better for it.

I would also like to relate another little insight I have regarding these weight charts. Almost every overweight patient seems to think they fall into the "large frame" category. This just isn't so. Be honest with yourself. Determine which category you do fall into, and then choose the ideal weight accordingly. Don't automatically think you're a large-framed individual just because you're overweight. I know it's easier to contemplate a loss of say, only forty pounds as opposed to sixty pounds, but if what you really need to lose is sixty pounds, stop kidding yourself. Let's choose the really desirable weight for you instead of one that you think will be "O.K."

The *Super 500 Rapid Weight Loss Program* is so easy to follow and so quick, that there is no reason for you to kid yourself any longer. You may as well lose all those excess pounds, know that you are successful, and be proud of your achievement.

Now, before going to the next paragraph, please go to the appropriate desirable weight chart and determine the ideal weight for you.

How to Know When You'll Reach Your Goal

Just as it's important to know how many pounds to lose, it is also important to know when you will lose them. By setting your goals realistically, you will experience a certain satisfaction once they are achieved. Since the Super 500 Program is extremely rapid in producing weight loss, you

CHART 4-A: DESIRABLE WEIGHT FOR MEN WHO ARE PRESENTLY OVERWEIGHT

Height	Small Frame	Medium Frame	Large Frame
5'2"	118-125	123-135	132-149
5'3"	121-129	127-138	135-151
5'4"	125-133	130-143	138-156
5'5"	129-136	135-147	142-160
5'6"	132-142	137-153	146-167
5'7"	135-145	143-157	150-170
5'8"	140-150	146-161	155-175
5'9"	144-153	150-165	160-180
5'10"	148-158	154-170	164-185
5'11"	153-163	157-174	168-189
6'0"	156-167	162-180	173-194
6'1"	161-171	167-185	178-199
6'2"	163-174	173-191	183-204
6'3"	167-177	178-199	189-216
6'4"	171-180	187-205	196-225

CHART 4-B: DESIRABLE WEIGHT FOR WOMEN WHO ARE PRESENTLY OVERWEIGHT

Height	Small Frame	Medium Frame	Large Frame
4'10"	93-99	98-111	106-123
4'11"	96-104	101-114	108-126
5'0"	98-108	104-116	113-129
5'1"	103-111	107-119	115-132
5'2"	105-114	111-123	119-135
5'3"	108-116	113-125	121-138
5'4"	111-119	116-130	125-142
5'5"	115-123	120-134	129-147
5'6"	117-127	125-140	134-151
5'7"	122-131	128-143	137-154
5'8"	125-135	132-148	141-158
5'9"	130-140	136-151	145-163
5'10"	133-143	140-156	149-168
5'11"	138-149	145-159	153-175
6'0"	142-154	150-164	158-180

should have no fear that you won't lose the number of pounds desired. By the same token, since the Super 500 Program is enjoyable and easy to live with, you can put your mind at ease regarding any possible failure or backsliding.

The Super 500 Program is based on a twenty-one/seven-day schedule. By this I mean that twenty-one days in a row you will follow the Rapid Weight Reduction portion of the program, then, for seven days, you will maintain a three-meal-per-day regimen.

This alternation between rapid weight reduction and weight maintenance provides a great degree of variety in addition to what is already included in the program. Since you are already aware of your present weight and have already determined your ideal weight, the only thing to do now is subtract your ideal weight from your present weight and determine the number of pounds you wish to lose. Next, you should consult Chart 4-C or Chart 4-D to determine how many pounds you will lose at the end of twenty-one days on the program.

For instance, let's assume that you are a man, 6'2" tall, of medium frame, and should weigh between 173 and 191 pounds. Let us also assume that you have decided you would do well at a weight almost in the middle of that range, i.e., you are trying to achieve an ideal weight of 182 pounds. For the purposes of this illustration, pretend that your job requires heavy physical labor. By going to Chart 4-D for men and looking up your present weight of 212 pounds, you will immediately see that at the end of twenty-one days, you will have lost 29 ½ pounds. In only a three-week span, you will have attained your ideal weight (or within a pound or two of it). At that time, you should go on the seven-day maintenance program as outlined in Chapter 8. Don't forget; what we assumed here was that you were doing heavy physical labor in your job, so we went to the maximum weight loss table.

Now, on the other hand, assume you had a sedentary occupation or perhaps were retired and rarely involved yourself in any physical activity. In that event, I would have suggested you go to Chart 4-C for men, and if you look at that section now, you will see that in twenty-one days you would

CHART 4-C: The Super 500 Twenty-One-Day Weight Loss Schedule

MINIMUM WEIGHT LOSSES

Directions: Find your present weight within the present weight ranges of the appropriate column. Read the *least* amount of weight which will be lost in twenty-one days to the right of your present weight range.

MEN			WOMEN	
PRESENT WEIGHT RANGES		MINIMUM WEIGHT LOSS IN 21 DAYS	PRESENT WEIGHT RANGES	MINIMUM WEIGHT LOSS IN 21 DAYS
141-150	7		91-100	2¼
151-160	7¾		101-110	3
161-170	8¾		111-120	3¾
171-180	9½		121-130	4½
181-190	10½		131-140	5½
191-200	11¼		141-150	6¼
201-210	12		151-160	7
211-220	13		161-170	7¾
221-230	13¾		171-180	8½
231-240	14½		181-190	9¼
241-250	15½		191-200	10
251-260	16¼		201-210	10¾
261-270	17¼		211-220	11¾
271-280	18		221-230	12½
281-290	18¾		231-240	13¼
291-300	19¾		241-250	14
301-310	20½		251-260	14¾
311-320	21¼		261-270	15½
321-330	22¼		271-280	16¼
331-340	23		281-290	17
341-350	23¾		291-300	18

have lost 13 pounds. This is the minimum weight loss possible, while following the program, for an individual who does little more than sit around all day and eat. In any event, at the end of twenty-one days you would have lost the 13 pounds, but would not have achieved your weight loss goal. At this point, you would go on to the Triple Threat Program

CHART 4-D: The Super 500 Twenty-One-Day Weight Loss Schedule

MAXIMUM WEIGHT LOSS

Directions: Find your present weight within the present weight ranges of the appropriate column. Read the *most* amount of weight which will be lost in twenty-one days and to the right of your present weight range.

MEN		WOMEN	
141-150	18	91-100	9
151-160	19¾	101-110	10½
161-170	21¼	111-120	12
171-180	23	121-130	13½
181-190	24½	131-140	15
191-200	26¼	141-150	16½
201-210	27¾	151-160	18
211-220	29½	161-170	19½
221-230	31	171-180	21
231-240	32½	181-190	22½
241-250	34¼	191-200	24
251-260	35¾	201-210	25½
261-270	37½	211-220	27
271-280	39	221-230	28½
281-290	40½	231-240	30
291-300	42¼	241-250	31½
301-310	43¾	251-260	33
311-320	45½	261-270	34½
321-330	47	271-280	36
331-340	48¾	281-290	37½
341-350	50¼	291-300	39

for seven days, after which you would have lost another two to five pounds. At the end of the seven-day Triple Threat Program, you would once again return to the 500 Program for an additional twenty-one days.

As you can see by the chart, the additional twenty-one day program would have given you another 13-pound loss. This, coupled with the first 13 pounds, plus the 2 to 5 pounds you will have lost on the interim program, would have produced the ideal amount of weight loss, and you would have achieved your desirable weight. By then you would have returned to a normal dietary intake, your energy levels would have increased and you would be more active on a day-to-day basis.

Knowing when you will achieve your weight loss is extremely important, since it allows you to prepare yourself for your slenderness. Since it is virtually impossible to lose less or more weight than indicated on the tables, your present or starting weight may indicate that you have to utilize the twenty-one-day program more than once. This should be of little concern. As I have said previously, the twenty-one-day Super 500 Program is enjoyable and satisfying, produces minimal amounts of stress and anxiety, and can be used over and over again until you attain the weight that's ideal for you.

Although there is considerable variation between the minimum and maximum weight loss possible on the twenty-one-day program, you will undoubtedly fall closer to the maximum weight loss since the minimum is based, as I have said before, on an individual who does absolutely nothing. If you desire to increase the rapidity with which you lose weight, I have included Chapter 8 specifically for you. By utilizing the recommendations in Chapter 8, you will find yourself melting away those pounds faster than you thought possible; faster even than is indicated by the maximum weight loss charts. But enough of this. You can determine whether or not you wish to increase the speed with which you lose weight when the time arrives.

How Margaret S. Dropped 54 Pounds Using the Super "500" Approach

When Margaret first decided to lose weight, she was fifty-four years old. She weighed 194 pounds and was 5'6" tall. After I discussed her weight loss with her, Margaret decided that 140 pounds would be ideal for her. She couldn't decide whether she was of medium or large frame, and therefore picked the highest weight desirable in the medium frame category as her goal.

In all honesty, Margaret did have a large frame and she could have carried a few more pounds without difficulty. In any event, she chose 140 pounds as her goal, so it was imperative that she achieve it. Margaret was not working at the time she began her program, and her only activities were those of a housekeeper and wife. I agree that there is a considerable amount of activity necessary to keep a house going, but to my mind I didn't feel Margaret would achieve weight loss in the maximum category. She fooled me! Margaret undertook two twenty-one-day programs with one seven-day interim period. When she completed her total program less than two months after initiating it, Margaret had lost a total of 54 pounds and looked super.

I recall once asking Margaret how she was losing faster than anticipated. She replied that the Super 500 Program had permitted her to eat more food than she really wanted. She had, therefore, voluntarily cut back on the quantity of satisfiers she consumed.

She knew that she would have lost the weight in almost the same amount of time had she eaten the full amount of satisfiers, but Margaret stated that the satisfiers were too filling, that she felt stuffed, and therefore had decided she didn't need all that food. She reduced the amounts accordingly.

She told me that she never felt hungry while on the program and that if she had felt that she was losing energy, she would have forced herself to take the extra amounts of satisfiers as recommended. Fortunately though, the quantities that Margaret consumed were more than adequate for her needs and she did not require more.

By this simple alteration of the program, Margaret had been able to by-pass the maximum weight loss expected even for a very, very active person. Along with these factors, Margaret, in addition to her normal housework chores and the reduction in the quantity of satisfiers, also took advantage of the "Metabolic Bath." (Please see Chapter 14.)

You can do the same! By taking a few minutes to make some small modifications in your program as outlined, you will find you can increase your weight loss dramatically.

How to Give Yourself a Chance to Reap the Rewards

I have had a number of patients come to me and ask why they could not continue on with the twenty-one-day program. They felt satisfied and were enjoying themselves, and at the same time were losing weight rapidly. They couldn't understand why they had to go over to the seven-day interim period.

Since you may find yourself wanting to continue on the twenty-one-day program because you are feeling so good, let me stress the importance of using the interim period appropriately.

The large amount of weight you will be losing during the first three weeks of your Super 500 Program must be consolidated. By that I mean that your body must adapt to its new lowered weight: it must be given a chance to "balance out." Please don't think of this as some unnecessary delay, as I assure you it is essential. I know that once you start to see those pounds melt away, you'll want to continue with the original program; however, I strongly suggest that you benefit from my experience with other patients, and utilize the seven-day interim program. Not only will this seven-day alteration permit your body to adapt to its new lower weight; it will also give you the opportunity to adapt psychologically to your slenderness.

At the same time, the change in food consumption will act as a variable. You will find that by eating more, during this one week section of the program, you will become remotivated to once again go back onto the twenty-one-day program if you require an additional loss of weight. Please don't yield to the temptation to continue on with the twenty-one-day program beyond the three-week period. Doing this may lessen your resolve and cause you to stop short of your weight loss goal. Reap the rewards you're entitled to; enjoy yourself for one week before continuing on to achieve your final weight.

Enjoying the Interim

The seven-day interim program is designed to accomplish several things. First, as I mentioned above, it's intended to allow your body to adapt to its new lower weight. Physiologically the loss of excess weight puts a certain amount of strain on your homeostatic mechanisms. By this I mean that it will take your body some time to adjust to the newer, lower requirements produced by your lighter weight. In addition, the seven-day interim program also gives you a breather: a chance to recoup your motivation and to enjoy the weight loss already achieved. For seven days you will be able to eat more food in a greater variety than while you were on the twenty-one-day portion of the program. I am sure you will find that variety truly is the spice of life, and this seven-day interim will be extremely enjoyable.

Be assured that I too want you to lose as much weight, as quickly as possible, but I also want you to have a good time while doing it. Finally then, I urge you to take advantage of the seven-day interim program. Give yourself a chance to enjoy its rewards.

CHAPTER 5

HOW TO USE PRE-PROGRAMMING FOR FASTEST RESULTS

You are now ready to lose those excess pounds. You know precisely how much you need to lose, and when you'll lose it. Simply follow the directions in the next section, and in twenty-one days you'll be a new, slender individual.

The Interlocking Directorate and How It Works

In the following pages you will find seven daily menus. Each menu has been designed to provide a specific number of calories. In addition, the foods permitted have been combined in a prescribed manner.

Each daily menu stands by itself. Do not try to combine one breakfast with another day's lunch or dinner. Do not substitute a particular satisfier with one from another day. If you do this, the program will not work. The food permitted on any one day can be eaten as you like, but always keep at least three hours between any particular meal and any satisfier. If you eat a meal within three hours of a satisfier or another meal, you will restrict your weight loss.

Remember, eat only the foods listed for the particular

day, and keep the meals and satisfiers separated by at least three hours. That's all there is to it.

Once you have completed the first week on the program, return to Day One and proceed through the seven daily menus once again. Do this one final time to reach the end of your twenty-one-day program. At that point, follow the instructions in Chapter 8.

Day One Breakfast

MENU

O.J. Bubbly
Fried Egg
Buttered Toast
Black Coffee or Tea

O.J. Bubbly

Into a tall glass (12 oz.) pour 4 oz. unsweetened orange juice, (preferably fresh squeezed). Add 1 ice cube and stir till melted. Fill remainder of the glass with chilled club soda or "highly carbonated" mineral water.

Fried Egg

Heat fry pan over *low* heat, add small pat of butter. When butter melts, wipe out excess with paper towel. Slide egg gently into pan. Add 1 tsp. tap water and cover. After 1-2 minutes remove cover and turn egg if desired. Serve on heated plate.

Buttered Toast

Use ½ slice bread of your choice (although dark breads are preferred), spread small amount of butter (approximately ½ tsp.) over toast and serve.

Black Coffee or Tea

May be taken as desired. If you will be drinking only one cup, be sure that it is strong.

NOTES

I think you'll enjoy the O.J. Bubbly. It is refreshing and has a unique taste. If you are using mineral water, be sure it is "highly carbonated," otherwise the drink will seem *flat.* Sip the drink slowly, and don't eat for at least 15 minutes.

Small or medium sized eggs are less fattening than large and extra large. You might get into the habit of using the smaller sizes. Doing so will help you maintain your lowered weight later on.

Toast that is "burned," although it contains the same number of calories, seems to be more satisfying or filling than lightly toasted bread. Whole wheat bread, toasted twice, is especially tasty. Try it, you may like it.

Your weight this morning is your "Starting Weight" for the purposes of this program. Each morning you should weigh yourself prior to eating anything, and at exactly the same time each day (even on weekends). This is the only way to get an accurate picture of your weight loss.

Dining Out?

Prepare your own O.J. Bubbly by ordering a small orange juice and a half glass of carbonated soda water. Pour ⅔ of the O.J. into the water. Voila! O.J. Bubbly "restaurant style."

Most restaurants cook with excessive fats. Either order a poached egg, or if you desire fried, order your toast "dry." In any event, when eating out you should always request "butter on the side." This way you can judge how much to use. Don't overdo it—butter is extremely high in calories.

*****

Day One Mid-Morning Satisfier

Mint Pineapple Frost

In a blender, combine 12 oz. of chilled apricot nectar, 6 oz. of pineapple juice, icy cold; and ½ tsp. of peppermint extract. Blend at high speed until frothy. Pour over crushed ice in tall glasses and add a mint sprig if desired. This recipe makes 5 tall frosties, one glass equals one satisfier. Save the remainder for another day, or share it with others.

*****

Day One Lunch

MENU

Steaming Bouillon
Crisp Chef Salad
with
Dressing
Black Coffee or Tea

Steaming Bouillon

Bring 1½ cups of water to a boil, add 1 bouillon cube and stir till dissolved. Beef or chicken flavored bouillon may be used. If you have some homemade broth available, you may use this if you remove all visible fat. See NOTES section.

Crisp Chef Salad

Wash, pat dry, and tear 1 cup of fresh greens (lettuce, escarole, kale) into bite-sized pieces. Place in a large bowl, add 2 tbs. of French or Italian dressing. Toss to coat all the greens. Add ½ slice of boiled ham, ½ slice of rolled turkey, and ½ slice of American or Swiss cheese. Toss gently and serve.

Coffee or Tea

As desired.

NOTES

A steaming cup of broth or bouillon is an excellent start to any meal. There are essentially no calories in this flavorful treat, so you can have as much as you want. Because of the high content of sodium (salt) in commercial bouillon, you may be wise in not overdoing it. It will only increase your desire for liquids later on.

If you have home-made broth, you must remove the fat because it contains enormous amounts of calories. To do this you can place the broth in the refrigerator overnight, and then remove the hardened layer of fat with a spoon the next day. If the broth is freshly made, use a piece of brown paper (a portion of a shopping bag is fine) to absorb the fat floating on top. Another method is to add two or three ice cubes to the still warm broth, stir once and the fat will partially harden. You can then remove it with a ladle.

When adding salad dressing (or any high calorie item) to your meals, you must be accurate in the amounts used. Two tablespoons means two *level* tablespoons. Don't overdo it!

The meats and cheese permitted in the Chef Salad have been estimated according to what is normally available in most supermarkets. One slice is approximately ⅛" thick; use only ½ slice of each in your salad.

Dining Out?

Most restaurants serve commercially prepared broth or bouillon, and although these usually contain some added fat (just to make it look richer), it is OK to eat these. One serving is all that is permitted though.

Additionally, restaurant-style Chef Salads usually contain more meat, cheese and dressing than is permitted. You may do best by ordering the salad with the dressing on the side, and "hold the egg."

*****

Day One Mid-Afternoon Satisfier

Juicy Cooler

In a pitcher, combine a 6 oz. can of frozen grapefruit-orange juice concentrate with 1 cup of cold water and 1½ cups of ice cubes. Stir till ice is nearly melted. Add a dash of bitters if desired and 12 oz. of low calorie lemon-lime soda. Stir gently (so as to not remove the carbonation from the drink) and serve over ice. Makes 6 satisfiers.

*****

Day One Dinner

MENU

Tossed Green Salad
Beef Steak with Mushrooms
Buttered Asparagus Spears
Gelatin Dessert
Black Coffee or Tea

Tossed Green Salad

Use 1 cup of fresh greens (preferably spinach, mustard, or collard) torn into bite-size pieces and washed thoroughly. Toss together gently with 1 tb. of Italian salad dressing.

Beef Steak

In a small skillet, sprinkle approximately ¼ tsp. of salt. Place over medium high heat. When thoroughly heated, place a 4 oz. steak in the pan (rib eye is excellent). Cook until seared, turn once and leave cooking for 2-3 minutes. Add 4-6 oz. of canned or fresh mushroom slices that have been washed and dried after removing the steak to a serving dish. Add a dash or two of Soy Sauce, stir briskly until the mushrooms are heated through.

Spoon the mushrooms and whatever sauce is in the pan over the steak. Serve immediately.

Buttered Asparagus Spears

Use canned spears heated thoroughly in their own juices. Do not overcook. Remove and drain. Add 1 tsp. of butter and mix gently to coat. Serve immediately. Six to eight spears equal a serving.

Gelatin Dessert

Use any gelatin dessert of your choice and prepare according to package directions, but adding an extra ½ cup of water to the preparation. Chill till firm and serve in dessert dish. Three heaping tablespoons of dessert are equal to a serving.

Black Coffee or Tea

As desired.

NOTES

The fresh greens recommended for this evening's salad are extremely good sources of iron (a necessary blood-building element). Mustard and collard greens contain more iron and are less expensive than is spinach. You can save some money and still get this important mineral.

A juicy steak smothered with mushrooms is the favorite of many. I have recommended a rib eye steak because it is easily trimmed of excess fat. Whatever cut of beef you enjoy, be sure to remove all visible fat *before* cooking.

Dining Out?

No need to alter your meal if you're eating at a restaurant. Just be sure not to overdo it—4 oz. of steak are all that's permitted.

*****

Day One Late-Evening Satisfier

Strawberries alá Creme

Crush ¼ cup of fresh strawberries, mix with ¼ cup of whipped dessert topping, ¼ cup of 2 percent yogurt, and non-caloric sweetener equal to 1 tbs. sugar.

Divide 2 cups of fresh strawberries into 4 equal parts, wash and slice in halves. Place these in 4 sherbet dishes and top with the crushed strawberry mixture. UMMM! Delicious.

Each dish equals one satisfier.

*****

Day Two Breakfast

MENU

*Hot Cereal
with
Milk and Sugar
Black Coffee or Tea*

Hot Cereal

Any cooked cereal you enjoy may be eaten. Be sure it is unsweetened though. Prepare it with *water*, not milk, in accordance with package directions. One half cup is permitted.

Milk and Sugar

Skim milk is preferred, but 1 percent or 2 percent fat milk is permissible. Use ½ cup if skim; 3 oz. if 1 percent or 2 percent fat. One level teaspoon of sugar is permitted. Any non-caloric sugar substitute may be used if you wish to restrict your intake of calories.

Black Coffee or Tea

May be taken as desired. If you will be drinking only one cup, be sure it is *strong*.

NOTES

This morning the scale should already show a weight loss. Even though fat is being quickly removed from your body, the weight lost this morning is primarily water (interstitial fluids). It will take several days before the actual fat reduction starts to be reflected on your scale.

Hot cereal usually "sticks to the ribs." Although in the past you probably ate a larger amount, ½ cup is more than sufficient if eaten *slowly*. Don't rush your meals.

Dining Out?

You shouldn't have any problem obtaining the above breakfast in a restaurant. Don't be embarrassed to ask for what you want. Remember—the customer is always right.

When eating hot cereal in a restaurant, try to gauge the amount you eat. Oatmeal, for instance, is usually served in an 8 oz. (1 cup) bowl. Leave half the cereal (or request a half-size portion) and you will have no problem.

Be sure to ask for skim milk. Every calorie counts.

*****

Day Two Mid-Morning Satisfier

Apple Cooler

In a pitcher, combine 2 cups of apple juice, 12 oz. of apricot nectar, ¼ cup of lemon juice and three dashes of bitters. Pour 21 oz. of club soda into the juice mixture. Stir gently and serve over ice. Makes 8 satisfiers.

*****

Day Two Lunch

MENU

Sweet and Creamy Bagels
Fresh Melon
Black Coffee or Tea

Sweet and Creamy Bagels

Toast ½ bagel. Spread with 1 tb. softened cream cheese and then sprinkle with a small amount of cinnamon. Place two wedges of canned or fresh peaches on top and then add 3 thin slices of banana. Serve with:

Fresh Melon

⅙ of a cantaloupe or honeydew.

Black Coffee or Tea

As desired.

NOTES

Don't be misled by the fact that only ½ of a bagel is permitted for lunch today. The cream cheese and banana slices are excellent foods for producing that "full" feeling. Because of their high fat content these foods remain in the stomach longer than most, thereby preventing hunger pangs and growling stomachs. I think you'll be pleased with the way this lunch satisfies that "sweet tooth."

Dining Out?

Almost every restaurant serves some form of "Dieter's Delite." These usually consist of a hamburger pattie, cottage cheese and some fruit. A good restaurant substitute for today's lunch is a scoop of cottage cheese (creamed is OK) and some mixed fruits. A few slices (2) of Melba toast may also be eaten, if desired. No hamburger allowed.

Another possible restaurant meal would consist of Date/Nut bread toasted and spread with cream cheese: a true taste delight.

Of course you can have a toasted bagel with cream cheese instead if that's what you want. Eat either ½ bagel and have a slice of melon, or have a whole bagel and eliminate the fruit.

*****

Day Two Mid-Afternoon Satisfier

Sweet and Tangy Sherbet

Combine ½ cup sugar, 1½ tsp. unflavored gelatin, and a pinch of salt in a saucepan. Stir in 1 cup of low-cal Cranberry Juice Cocktail. Warm over medium heat while stirring, till the sugar dissolves. Remove from heat and stir in another cup of Cranberry Juice Cocktail and the juice of ½ lemon. Freeze. When almost firm beat with an electric mixer until smooth. Re-freeze till completely firm. Makes 6 satisfiers.

*****

Day Two Dinner

MENU

Tomatoes Vinaigrette
Spicy Ham Broil
Black Coffee or Tea

Tomatoes Vinaigrette

Slice two medium-sized tomatoes into thin slices. In a separate bowl, combine 1 tsp. salad oil, 2 tbs. vinegar, ¼ tsp. oregano, and ¼ tsp rosemary or sage. Mix until the herbs are completely moistened. Pour over tomato slices. Serves 2.

Spicy Ham Broil

Cook a 10 oz. package of frozen asparagus spears according to directions. While cooking, toast 4 slices of white bread, and spread with mustard. Place 1 slice of boiled ham on each piece of toast. Place an equal number of asparagus spears on each ham-topped toast, and sprinkle a mixture of shredded Swiss cheese and chopped scallions on top of all. Use approximately 2 oz. of Swiss cheese to 2 tbs. of chopped scallions. Broil just until the cheese melts. Serves 4.

Black Coffee or Tea

As desired.

NOTES

The tomatoes vinaigrette will taste better if you can prepare the oil/vinegar combination beforehand. Let the herbal flavors mix by themselves in the refrigerator for an hour or two and you'll be surprised at how delicious this tomato salad will taste.

Some patients have found that adding a tablespoon or two of chopped pimiento to the cheese and scallion topping increases the flavor. You might want to try this.

Dining Out?

An open-faced ham Reuben sandwich is a good substitute for tonight's dinner. If ham is unavailable and corned beef must be used, be sure it is trimmed of all visible fat. No salad is permitted though, because the restaurant sandwich will contain more meat and cheese than is permitted in the home-cooked meal.

*****

Day Two Late-Evening Satisfier

Strawberry-Melon Parfait

Quarter 2½ cups of fresh strawberries and sprinkle with 1 tb.

of sugar. Mash together 1 large ripe banana, ½ cup of plain yogurt, 2 tsps. of sugar and a generous pinch of cinnamon.

Dice two cups of honeydew melon and arrange in 6 parfait dishes. Spoon half of the yogurt mixture over the diced melon. Top with the sweetened strawberries, then spoon the remaining yogurt mixture over all. Garnish with a sprinkle of cinnamon if desired. Makes 6 satisfiers.

*****

Day Three Breakfast

MENU

Sparkling Lemon Tonic
High Protein Crisp Cereal
with
Milk and Sugar
Black Coffee or Tea

Sparkling Lemon Tonic

Into a tall glass (12 oz.) squeeze the juice of ¼ of a large lemon. Gently fill with chilled club soda or sparkling mineral water by slowly pouring down the side of the glass. Do not stir!

High Protein Crisp Cereal

There are a number of protein fortified breakfast cereals. Be sure the one you choose does not contain any added sugar. Get into the habit of reading labels. Use ¾ cup dry cereal.

Milk

Skim milk is preferred, but 1 percent or 2 percent fat milk is permissible. Be sure it is icy cold before pouring on the cereal. Use ½ cup if skim, 3 oz. if 1 percent or 2 percent fat.

Sugar

One level teaspoon is permitted.

Black Coffee or Tea

May be taken as desired. If you will be drinking only one cup, be sure that it is *strong*.

NOTES

This morning's breakfast is quite light, but it will supply more than adequate nutrition without putting undue stress on your digestive system.

Don't forget—sip the tonic slowly and do not eat until at least 15 minutes after you've finished it.

Be sure to use exactly one level teaspoon of granulated sugar with your breakfast. You may want to use only a part of this amount on your cereal and the remainder in your coffee or tea. You can do the same with your milk allowance if desired.

When you weighed in this morning you should have noticed only a slight reduction in weight as compared to yesterday. This is normal. Your body is still retaining fluids and it will take several more days to notice the true weight loss. Don't be discouraged by your scale's failure to reflect the actual amount of fat already discarded.

Try to find some time this evening to luxuriate in the pleasures of the Metabolic Bath. (Chapter 8)

Dining Out?

Most restaurants maintain a basic inventory of dry cereals. If you are unable to obtain a high protein cereal, choose any *dry*, unsweetened cereal you enjoy. Generally, the individual serving sizes contain one ounce of cereal. This is comparable to a ¾ cup serving.

Be sure to use skim milk. If the restaurant you're eating in doesn't carry it, order a small glass of whole milk (8 oz.) and use it *all*. Then refrain from taking the mid-morning satisfier.

NOTE: If you frequent the same restaurant almost daily, I'm sure the proprietor would be happy to order the cereal you like, and also keep a quart of skim milk just for you. Ask. You have nothing to lose but extra pounds.

*****

Day Three Mid-Morning Satisfier

Creamy Banana Thick Shake

Cut one small banana into chunks. Freeze. When solidly frozen, combine with ½ cup skim milk, and non-caloric sweetener equal to 1 tb. sugar, in a blender. Blend until thick and creamy. Serve in an Old Fashioned glass with a pinch of cinnamon on top. Makes 1 satisfier.

*****

Day Three Lunch

MENU

Crunchy Garden Sandwich
Black Coffee or Tea

Crunchy Garden Sandwich

Mix ¼ cup of vinegar with 2 tbs. of water, 1 tsp. of dillweed, a dash of pepper, and 1 large unpeeled cucumber, thinly sliced. Allow flavors to mix in the refrigerator for one to two hours.

Spread 4 tsp. of butter on 4 slices of dark bread (pumpernickel is excellent). Top with drained cucumbers and a thinly sliced radish. Serves 4.

Black Coffee or Tea

As desired.

NOTES

The fresh clean taste of crunchy vegetables is invigorating. With today's lunch you might want to have a sliced tomato. No problem; enjoy.

Instead of butter, try mayo on the bread; you may find it enhances the flavor of the garden fresh vegetables. Not too much though; there are a lot of calories in both these spreads.

Dining Out?

Unless you're eating in a health food restaurant, you'll be hard put to find this sandwich on the menu. Instead, why not try a *small* mixed salad. Go easy on the dressing, and substitute two slices of Melba toast for the slice of bread.

*****

Day Three Mid-Afternoon Satisfier

Cola Café

Combine 1½ cups skim milk, 2 tbs. sugar, 2 tbs. instant coffee powder, and ¼ tsp. cinnamon in a blender. Blend well.

When ready to serve, add 16 oz. low-calorie cola soda. Stir gently so as to not let it lose its "head." Serve over ice. Makes 6 satisfiers.

*****

Day Three Dinner

MENU

Chicken Salad àla Parmesan
Black Coffee or Tea

Chicken Salad àla Parmesan

Combine 1 head of Romaine lettuce, torn into bite-sized pieces; 2 cups of cooked cubed chicken; and 2 tbs. of grated Parmesan cheese.

In a separate bowl, mix ⅔ cup low-calorie Italian salad dressing, 4 tsp. vinegar, ½ tsp. dry mustard, and ¼ tsp. Worcestershire sauce.

Add to salad and toss till salad is coated. Add 1 cup croutons and toss gently to mix. Makes 6 servings.

Black Coffee or Tea

As desired.

NOTES

I personally love this salad combination. Usually though, I use fresh escarole instead of Romaine. I like the tart, tangy taste.

I should tell you that I also use Romano cheese instead of Parmesan. Guess why?

Dining Out?

A chef salad "restaurant style" is an excellent substitute for this chicken salad. Go lightly on the dressing though.

*****

Day Three Late-Evening Satisfier

Lemon Puff

In a large bowl, dissolve a 3 oz. package of lemon flavored gelatin in 1 cup of boiling water. Add 2½ tbs. lemon juice (fresh is preferred, but bottled is OK) and ¾ cup of cold water. Stir well, then chill.

When the gelatin partially sets, add 2 egg whites to the gelatin mixture, and beat with an electric mixer until fluffy. Spoon into 8 pudding cups and chill until set.

In a saucepan, blend 1 tbs. of cornstarch and ½ cup of cold water. Add ½ cup of crushed blueberries and 2 tbs. of sugar to the cornstarch mixture. Cook over medium heat till mixture thickens. Stir constantly. Once the mixture thickens, cook for an additional 2 minutes. Remove from heat, add 1 cup of fresh whole blueberries, and ¼ tsp. of vanilla extract. Chill.

To serve, spoon generous amounts of the blueberry sauce over the lemon puff pudding. Makes 8 satisfiers.

*****

Day Four Breakfast

MENU

Sliced Apricots
Flaked Corn Cereal
with
Milk and Sugar
Black Coffee or Tea

Sliced Apricots

Chilled, canned apricots are delicious. Be sure to use a product that is unsweetened and packed in it's own juices, or is labelled "water pack." One half cup is permitted. Try to measure ¼ cup of fruit and ¼ cup of juice.

If you prefer fresh fruit, two whole apricots are permitted.

Flaked Corn Cereal

Corn or wheat flakes are recommended and a ¾ cup serving is permitted.

Milk and Sugar

½ cup skim milk or 3 oz. 1 percent or 2 percent fat. One level teaspoon granulated sugar.

Black Coffee or Tea

As desired.

NOTES

By this morning your body should be adjusting to the change in food intake. Most dieters report that a feeling of calmness comes over them about the fourth or fifth day of the program. This is primarily due to the program's ability to stabilize blood-sugar levels. Today's weigh-in should reflect additional pounds lost.

When fruit is permitted with dry cereal, you might enjoy mixing them together. Eliminate the sugar and you will lose even faster.

Dining Out?

I doubt if you'll find too many restaurants serving apricots, so you'll have to substitute chilled tomato juice. Order a small glass, perhaps with a squeeze of fresh lemon to give it a little added flavor. Don't add salt to it though—you don't want your body to retain excess fluids.

*****

Day Four Mid-Morning Satisfier

Orange Jubilee

Section 4 peeled oranges. Add 2 medium bananas already sliced, and 3 maraschino cherries that have been quartered. Toss gently and sprinkle with 2 tbs. shredded coconut. Makes 6 satisfiers.

*****

Day Four Lunch

MENU

Open-Faced Chicken Sandwich
Black Coffee or Tea

Open-Faced Chicken Sandwich

Mix together 2 tbs. flour, 1 tbs. sugar, 1 tsp. dry mustard, ½ tsp. salt, and ¼ tsp. pepper; stir in 2 egg yolks and ¾ cup skim milk. Cook over low heat while stirring. When thickened, add 3 tbs. vinegar; remove from heat and chill.

Spread 8 slices of dark bread with a small amount of the dressing, add 1 or 2 lettuce leaves and top with 1 slice of cooked chicken. Spread remaining dressing over all. Makes 8 sandwiches.

Black Coffee or Tea

As desired.

NOTES

When you taste this homemade dressing, I think you'll want to make it a part of your everyday fare. I find it to be so much better than commercially prepared mayonnaise. In the future, you can use it as an excellent substitute for mayo in all your recipes.

Dining Out?

Just order a sliced chicken sandwich with lettuce, mayo on the side. Then discard one slice of the bread and apply your own mayonnaise. About 1 tsp. is all you may use.

*****

Day Four Mid-Afternoon Satisfier

Georgia Ice/Florida Style

In a blender, combine 12 oz. of frozen peach slices with 1 cup of orange juice and 1 tbs. of freshly squeezed lemon juice. Blend well.

In a separate bowl, beat three egg whites to soft peaks. Add 3 tbs. sugar and beat until stiff. Fold into peach mixture and freeze till almost firm.

Beat again till smooth, then refreeze till firm. Spoon into sherbet dishes. Makes 8 satisfiers.

*****

Day Four Dinner

MENU

Super Chef Salad
Black Coffee or Tea

Super Chef Salad

In a large bowl combine 1 large head of Iceberg lettuce which has been torn into bite-size pieces, 2 ripe tomatoes cut in wedges, 3 hard-cooked eggs coarsely chopped, 1 small chopped onion, 4 slices of boiled ham that has been cut into thin strips, and 4 slices of Cheddar (or American) cheese, also cut into thin strips.

In a separate dish mix ¼ cup *each* of Italian and French salad dressings. Pour over salad and toss. Serves 8.

Black Coffee or Tea

As desired.

NOTES

Mixing French and Italian dressings together produces a unique flavor treat. Of course you can use either dressing by itself if you so desire, but I think you should experiment a little. Once you've tried these different combinations, you'll probably want to make them a part of your future life style.

The first time you have to prepare something new, you'll probably feel that it's not worth it. Once you get the hang of it and prepare these recipes from memory, you'll really enjoy making them.

Dining Out?

No problem! Just order a chef salad and ask for the dressing on the side. Use sparingly.

*****

Day Four Late-Evening Satisfier

Rice Pudding Especiale

In the top of a double boiler combine 1 cup skim milk, 2 cups water, ½ cup uncooked rice, ⅓ cup sugar, and ¼ tsp. salt. Cover and cook over boiling water for 1¼ hours. Stir frequently. Uncover, and cook till thickened (approximately 45 minutes). Remove from heat, stir in 1 tsp. vanilla extract and ¼ tsp. almond extract. Chill.

Beat 1 scant cup cottage cheese until smooth and fold into rice pudding. Stir till completely mixed. Serve in pudding dishes with grated orange peel to garnish. Makes 8 satisfiers.

*****

Day Five Breakfast

MENU

Lemon Tonic
Soft-Cooked Egg
Buttered Toast
Black Coffee or Tea

Lemon Tonic

See Day Three Breakfast.

Soft-Cooked Egg

Bring 1 cup of water, to which 1 tsp. salt has been added, to a boil. Gently lower a small or medium sized egg into the water with a spoon. Remove from heat and allow to cook for approximately 3 to 5 minutes, depending on your preference. Remove and plunge into cold water for a few seconds to stop the cooking process. Serve.

Buttered Toast

Use ½ slice bread of your choice (double toasted if you wish). Spread a small amount of butter on it (approximately ½ tsp.). If you would rather have a full slice of bread, just eliminate the butter.

Black Coffee or Tea

As desired.

NOTES

This morning's weight should once again be lower. By this time, the anxiety that normally accompanies a new dietary program should have been eliminated. You should be progressing calmly and with resolve toward your ideal weight. Don't let anyone upset you sufficiently to cause you to overeat.

Perhaps you weren't aware that most chefs consider egg boiling a "no-no." The proper way to prepare a soft- or hard-boiled egg is the way I've described earlier. Cooking an egg in boiling water toughens it.

The reason for the salt is to help prevent the egg shell from cracking. You'll never have this problem if you allow the egg to reach room temperature before you place it in the boiling water.

You'll have a hard time convincing a short-order cook that he shouldn't boil your egg. You'll do better to just order it the way you like it (3 minutes?) and ignore the fact that he cooked it the wrong way.

*****

Day Five Mid-Morning Satisfier

Pineapple-Raspberry Fizz

In a blender, combine 12 oz. of pineapple juice, 10 oz. of frozen raspberries, and ½ cup of water. Blend well, and strain. Slowly pour a quart bottle of low-calorie lemon-lime soda into the strained juice. Serve over crushed ice. Garnish with mint leaves. Makes 10 satisfiers.

*****

Day Five Lunch

MENU

*Crunchy-Creamy Cheese
Sandwich
Black Coffee or Tea*

Crunchy-Creamy Cheese Sandwich

Mash 1½ cups of cottage cheese with a fork. Mix in ½ cup chopped celery, ¼ cup shredded carrot, ¼ cup chopped radish, and ½ tsp. caraway seed.

Place 1 lettuce leaf on each of 6 slices of bread of your choice. Spread each slice with a generous amount of the cheese mixture. Makes 6 sandwiches.

Black Coffee or Tea

As desired.

NOTES

Because most dieters like to have a sandwich for their mid-day meal, I have included these on many days. A cup of bouillon or broth makes a good accompaniment to sandwich meals, and because it is so low in calories you can have it any time you wish.

Dining Out?

A large salad with a generous amount of dressing (blue Cheese?) is an excellent substitute for these homemade sandwiches. No bread is allowed though. The calorie content of the salad and the sandwich are almost equal. You don't want to overdo it.

*****

Day Five Mid-Afternoon Satisfier

Blueberry Ice

In a saucepan combine ¼ cup of sugar and ½ envelope of unflavored gelatin. Stir in 1 cup of water. Heat and stir until sugar dissolves.

Remove from heat; add ½ cup of water, 9 oz. of frozen blueberries and 3 tbs. of lemon juice. Freeze till almost firm, beat until smooth, and refreeze. Serve in sherbet dishes. Makes 8 satisfiers.

*****

Day Five Dinner

MENU

Pineapple Ham Medley
Black Coffee or Tea

Pineapple Ham Medley

In a large bowl, combine 8 oz. of drained, canned pineapple chunks; 4 slices of boiled ham, chopped; 1 cup seedless grapes; and 2 oz. mozzarella cheese, cut into strips.

In a blender, combine 1 cup cottage cheese, ½ cup skim milk, and ½ tsp. paprika. Blend till smooth.

Toss ham mixture with 1 head of lettuce that has been torn into bite-sized pieces. Serve in individual dishes with cottage cheese dressing over it. Makes 4 servings.

Black Coffee or Tea

As desired.

NOTES

This cottage cheese dressing is especially good with highly seasoned or flavorful salad combinations. If you wish to use it on a plain salad, you can add whatever seasonings will make it appetizing to you.

Dining Out?

Virginia Ham dinner without the potatoes will make an excellent restaurant substitute.

*****

Day Five Late-Evening Satisfier

Fruited Tea

In a saucepan, mix one 18 oz. can of pineapple juice, 2 cups of orange juice, 2 cups of water, 4 tsp. of instant tea powder, 1 tsp. allspice, and 1 stick of cinnamon. Bring to a boil, and simmer for 10 to 15 minutes. Strain. Makes 8 satisfiers.

*****

Day Six Breakfast

MENU

Fruit Cocktail
Puffed Wheat Cereal
with
Milk and Honey
Black Coffee or Tea

Fruit Cocktail

Canned fruit cocktail (any available brand), is recommended. Some enjoy this chilled, while others feel that the flavors are enhanced when it is eaten at room temperature. One half cup is permitted.

Puffed Wheat Cereal

Use ¾ cup *plain* unsweetened cereal.

Milk and Honey

One half cup skim, or 3 oz. 1 or 2 percent fat milk. For a taste treat mix 1 tsp. honey with the allowed milk before pouring it on the cereal. Don't forget—if you mix the fruit cocktail and cereal together, eliminate the honey.

Black Coffee or Tea

As desired.

NOTES

Your weight is continuing to drop. Each pound lost is primarily made up of excess fat, not just water. Today you should begin to feel a resurgence of energy. Most patients report that near the end of the first week of dieting, they feel so full of energy that they tackle jobs they've been postponing.

Either today or tomorrow, you should decide on some new physical activity. Walking, jogging, swimming, tennis, golf? All of these are excellent. Not only do these force you to lose faster, but they also make weight maintenance much easier.

Dining Out?

If you are unable to obtain fruit cocktail, substitute a small orange juice (6 oz.). Wheat flakes are an excellent substitute for the puffed cereal if it is unavailable. Although some restaurants serve honey, you may not be fortunate enough to eat at one of these. Substitute 1 tsp. pancake (maple?) syrup for the honey. The maple flavor complements the taste of wheat cereals. You may even enjoy it more than honey.

*****

Day Six Mid-Morning Satisfier

Mint Pineapple Frost

See Day One Mid-Morning Satisfier.

*****

Day Six Lunch

```
┌─────────────────────────────────────┐
│                MENU                 │
│                                     │
│         Ham Salad Sandwich          │
│         Black Coffee or Tea         │
└─────────────────────────────────────┘
```

Ham Salad Sandwich

Spread the insides of a frankfurter roll with prepared mustard. Using 2 slices of thinly sliced boiled ham, roll the following salad mixture inside (jelly roll fashion):

¼ cup shredded lettuce

½ tb. French salad dressing

1 dill pickle, chopped

Place in bun and heat if desired. Makes one sandwich.

Black Coffee or Tea

As desired.

NOTES

These sandwiches are fast and easy. Some patients make them using "Bavarian" style sauerkraut instead of the salad mix. If you don't mind skipping this afternoon's satisfier, add a slice of Swiss cheese on top of the sandwich before heating. This makes a pretty good "mock" Reuben.

Dining Out?

A frankfurter on a bun, with sauerkraut if you like, is a good substitute. A small green salad on the side with only a "smidgen" of French dressing is also permissible.

*****

Day Six Mid-Afternoon Satisfier

Creamy Banana Thick Shake

See Day Three Mid-Morning Satisfier.

*****

Day Six Dinner

MENU

Georgia Style Chicken
Black Coffee or Tea

Georgia Style Chicken

Mix together 1 oz. softened Neufchatel cheese, 2 tbs. mayonnaise, a pinch each of crushed thyme and basil leaves. Add ¼ lb. cooked, cubed chicken; 4 oz. canned, diced peaches; and ¼ cup chopped celery. Serve on crisp lettuce leaves. Makes 1 serving.

Black Coffee or Tea

As desired.

NOTES

The chopped peaches in this chicken salad really enhance the flavor. If you like, you can also add green pepper to the salad for additional crunchiness.

Dining Out?

The typical "Dieter's Delite," consisting of a small hamburger pattie, cottage cheese, and some canned fruit, is a good substitute for Georgia Style Chicken. It doesn't taste as good, but it's close enough calorie-wise.

*****

Day Six Late-Evening Satisfier

Strawberry Shake

In a blender, combine 1½ cups skim milk, 2 tbs. sugar, a dash of cinnamon, and 2 cups frozen, unsweetened strawberries. Blend until smooth, and serve immediately. Makes 5 satisfiers.

*****

Day Seven Breakfast

MENU

Fresh Grapefruit
Poached Egg
Toast
Black Coffee or Tea

Fresh Grapefruit

One half of a large, juicy, pink or white grapefruit is permitted. A light sprinkling of *salt* will enhance the flavor. Don't overdo it though.

Poached Egg

If you don't have an egg poacher, you can still do an adequate job by bringing ½ cup water, with ½ tsp. vinegar added, to a boil in a small frypan. Reduce heat and gently slide a small or medium egg into the water. Try stirring the water just before putting the egg in. The swirling movement tends to prevent the egg white from separating. Simmer for 3 to 5 minutes as desired. Serve on toast.

Toast

One slice only. No butter.

Black Coffee or Tea

As desired.

NOTES

You must decide what physical activity you want to take part in by this evening. Don't put this off! Even a 15-minute walk after dinner will be of enormous benefit in assisting the body to continue ridding itself of excess fat. The physical activity need not be strenuous—it's the movement that counts.

Dining Out?

You should have no trouble with today's breakfast. If grapefruit is unavailable, a small 6 oz. glass of chilled, unsweetened, grapefruit juice is an excellent substitute.

*****

Day Seven Mid-Morning Satisfier

Cola Cafe

See Day Three Mid-Afternoon Satisfier.

*****

Day Seven Lunch

MENU

Salmon Salad
Black Coffee or Tea

Salmon Salad

In a large mixing bowl, combine a 7½ oz. can of pink salmon, drained, boned and flaked; ½ cup mayonnaise; 2 tbs. finely chopped radishes; 2 tbs. chopped scallions (green onions); 1 tsp. soy sauce; and 1 tsp. freshly squeezed lemon juice. Mix well and spread evenly over 8 slices of well-toasted rye or pumpernickel bread. Top each sandwich with one slice of tomato. Makes 8 sandwiches.

Black Coffee or Tea

As desired.

NOTES

Today's lunch is really a taste treat. Some patients prepare the salmon salad the night before. They say that keeping it in the refrigerator overnight enhances the flavor.

If you would like a large dill or sour pickle with your sandwich, go ahead, and enjoy.

I hope you've also noticed that *pink* salmon is called for in the recipe. This is because it contains fewer calories than the red varieties.

An enjoyable variation is achieved if you replace the radishes with water chestnuts, chopped fine.

Dining Out?

There are three alternatives that can be substituted for today's lunch. They are:

1) Tuna Salad

2) Shrimp Salad

3) Chicken Salad

Whichever you choose, specify "open-faced," (on one slice of bread). Restaurant salads are very high in calories, so you might ask them to "go light on the mayo."

*****

Day Seven Mid-Afternoon Satisfier

Georgia Ice/Florida Style

See Day Four Mid-Afternoon Satisfier.

*****

Day Seven Dinner

MENU

Deviled Ham Sandwich
Black Coffee or Tea

Deviled Ham Sandwich

In a large bowl combine 1 egg, ⅓ cup skim milk, ½ cup bread crumbs, and ¼ cup chopped scallions. Add 2½ cups cooked ground ham. Mix well. Make into 6 patties, and brown over low heat in a large frypan. Place one pattie on half a well-toasted English muffin. Top with a mixture of chopped cucumbers and radishes. Spread with horseradish sauce. Makes 6 sandwiches.

Black Coffee or Tea

As desired.

NOTES

These sandwiches go especially well with pickled cucumbers and onions. You can prepare this side dish by thinly slicing 2 unpeeled cucumbers and 1 large onion. Place in a large bowl and cover with vinegar. Add pickling spices if desired. Let set in the refrigerator for at least 3 hours for best flavor. You can have as much of this as you like; it's very low in calories.

Dining Out?

A plain ¼ lb. hamburger is close in calories. Do without the bun and have a salad on the side. One tablespoon of dressing (your choice) is permitted.

*****

Day Seven Late-Evening Satisfier

Fruited Tea

See Day Five Late-Evening Satisfier.

*****

Hints on How to Do It Yourself

As I mentioned previously, it will be better for you and you will probably be more successful, if you follow the dietary program as I've outlined it in the previous pages. I realize, however, that some individuals do not like all foods, and perhaps some of the foods I've included in the seven daily menus are among them.

This is why I am including, in the following section, a list of foods that you can choose from to design your own daily menus. Be very careful, however, when you attempt to do this. It will take some time and concentration on your part to put together meals and daily menus that will produce the desired weight losses. Don't approach the design of these meals lightly. You will have to be extremely conscientious in picking the proper foods in the proper combinations if you wish to succeed.

If you are designing your own meals, you will be restricted in the particular satisfiers you can use. Because each meal in the seven daily menus includes specified quantities as well as preparation procedures, I have been able to include some high-calorie satisfiers. Unfortunately, when you design your own meals this cannot be done.

If you wish to be successful and lose those unwanted pounds, you must limit your satisfiers to:

A) Juicy Cooler—see Day One Mid-Afternoon Satisfier.

B) Strawberry Melon Parfait—see Day Two Late-Evening Satisfier.

C) Blueberry Ice—see Day Five Mid-Afternoon Satisfier.

The Juicy Cooler is lowest in calories and should be used most often. If you should find that on certain days you wish to design your own meals, you must restrict yourself to the above satisfiers. On the other days, if you will be eating the foods recommended in one of the seven daily menus, you may eat the satisfiers listed for those days.

In no event, however, should you mix and match, i.e., taking meals you've designed for yourself and incorporating them into the recommended menus. If you are determined to design your own meals, you must design the complete daily intake. Breakfast, lunch, dinner and three satisfiers from the above list must be formulated. Any alteration from this regimen and you may find yourself gaining weight instead of losing it.

Formulating Your Meals

In addition to three satisfiers which may be chosen from the above list, you must design three meals incorporating the following kinds and quantities of food.

Food	Quantity (in servings)
(A) Meat	5
(B) Fruit	2
(C) Fat	1
(D) Milk	1
(E) Bread	1
(F) Required Vegetable	1
(G) Vegetable as desired	2
(H) Free choices	4

Each of these food categories is listed below. The following example shows how you can design your own meal patterns. You are by no means restricted to following this particular example. You may eat the foods listed, in any order or combination that best suits you. Be certain, however, that you do not eat larger quantities than permitted.

Additionally, you must remember to keep your meals and satisfiers separated by at least three (3) hours. If you do not, you will inhibit your weight loss.

Good Luck!

A Typical Daily Meal Pattern Using the Above Listed Quantities of Food and Food Categories Listed Below

Food Categories

(A)(B)(C)(D)(E)(F)(G)(H)

Breakfast;

	(A)	(B)	(C)	(D)	(E)	(F)	(G)	(H)
½ cup tomato juice		1						
1 egg, poached	1							
1 slice bread, toasted					1			
½ tsp. butter			½					
½ cup skim milk				½				
coffee or tea, as desired								1

✳✳✳✳✳

Mid-Morning Satisfier
Juicy Cooler

✳✳✳✳✳

Lunch

1 cup beef bouillon				1
1 cup tossed salad, with			1	
1 tbs. blue cheese dressing	1	½		
½ cup skim milk			½	
1 small orange	1			
coffee or tea, as desired				1

*****

Mid-Afternoon Satisfier
   Blueberry Ice

*****

Dinner

3 oz. beef steak	3		
¼ cup green peas		½	
¼ cup cooked carrots		½	
1 small apple	1		
coffee or tea, as desired			1

*****

Late-Evening Satisfier
   Strawberry Melon
      Parfait

TOTAL   5 2 1 1 1 1 2 4

FOOD CATEGORIES

(A) Meat: (includes meat, fish, poultry, cheese, and eggs)

   Cheese—American, Swiss, Cheddar: 1 slice or 1
         oz.

   Cottage, uncreamed: ¼ cup

Cold Cuts—Bologna, Lunch loaf, Minced ham,
    Salami: 1 slice

Eggs—Prepared in any manner without added
    fat: 1 medium

Fish—Cod, halibut, trout, etc.: 1 oz. cooked
    Lobster, crabmeat: ¼ cup
    Sardines: 3 medium
    Shrimp, clams, oysters: 5 small
    Tuna, salmon: ¼ cup

Frankfurter—1
Meat—beef, chicken, ham, lamb, pork, turkey,
    veal: 1 oz. cooked.

(B) Fruit:
    Apple, 1
    Banana, ½ small
    Blueberries, ⅔ cup
    Cantaloupe, ¼
    Grapefruit, ½ small
    Grapefruit Juice, ½ cup
    Orange, 1 small
    Orange Juice, ½ cup
    Peach, 1 medium
    Pear, 1 small
    Plums, 2 medium
    Strawberries, 1 cup

(C) Fat:
    Bacon, crisp, 1 slice
    Butter or margarine, 1 tsp.
    Cream Cheese, 1 tbs.
    French or Italian Salad Dressing, 1 tbs.
    Mayonnaise, 1 tsp.
    Oils or shortening, 1 tsp.

(D) Milk:
    Whole milk, not permitted
    Skim milk, 1 cup
    1 or 2 percent fat milk, ½ cup

(E) Bread: (includes all grain, and starchy foods)
White, rye, whole wheat, 1 slice
Biscuit, 1 small
English muffin, ½
Frankfurter or Hamburger bun, ½
Melba toast, 4 slices

Cereal:
Cooked, ½ cup
Flaked or puffed, ¾ cup

Crackers:
Saltines, 5 (2″ square)
Noodles/Spaghetti/Rice/Grits:
½ cup, cooked

Potato:
1 boiled or baked, white. Mashed, ½ cup

(F) Required Vegetable: (½ cup cooked, or raw)
Beets, Carrots, Onions, Green Peas, Squash,
Turnip

**(G) Vegetable as desired: (any amount desired at
one time)**
Asparagus
Green Beans
Broccoli
Cabbage
Cauliflower
Celery
Cucumbers
Escarole
Greens: all kinds
Lettuce
Mushrooms
Green Pepper
Radishes
Sauerkraut
Tomatoes
Vegetable Juice Cocktail

(H) Free Choices (any amount at one sitting)
    Broth or Bouillon
    Coffee or Tea
    Low Calorie Gelatin
    Lemon
    Mustard
    Non-Caloric Sweetener
    Pepper and Spices
    Dill or Sour Pickles
    Vinegar

PLEASE NOTE: The above *Food Category List* may not contain some of the foods you normally eat. These foods were eliminated because, unless they are eaten in the proper combination with other foods on the list, they will prevent you from losing weight.

Since the Rapid Weight Loss portion of the program lasts only twenty-one days (and you'll be able to eat any food you like during the seven-day interim period) you shouldn't have too many problems designing a satisfactory meal schedule.

CHAPTER 6

COUNTDOWN:
ONLY 21 DAYS TO SLENDERNESS

Right now, right this very moment, you have all the necessary tools and information to begin your *Super 500 Rapid Weight Loss Program*. Don't put it off! Too many people procrastinate when it's time to lose weight. Making elaborate plans as to when you will start on your program only postpones the inevitable. Right this minute, you should begin to lose those unwanted pounds. The sooner you start, the sooner you'll finish. Telling yourself that you'll begin on Monday (or any other day besides today) is nothing more than a "cop-out." Why let yourself find a dozen excuses for not beginning this very instant?

You know you want to look good, be slender, and enjoy life. Don't fall for the psychological trap of postponing what must be done. I have heard any number of excuses; excuses that, on the surface at least, sounded feasible. Let me just list a few; then, if you find yourself thinking the same way, you will be able to change your reluctance to begin dieting into excitement and motivation to becoming slender.

"The weekends are always hardest. I'll wait till the kids go back to school (or my spouse goes back to work, or my mother-in-law goes home, etc."

"I can't start right this minute, I have to go to this special function (tonight, tomorrow night, etc.) and I'll have to eat what they serve."

"Next week would be best. It'll give me a chance to get ready."

"We're going on vacation. I'll start when we get back."

"I have company coming. I can't just stop everything and think about losing weight."

I think you get the idea. Every overweight individual has some excuse for not starting **now**. I even had a patient tell me that she had too much food (and goodies) in the house. She'd have to finish them up first (or else they'd go bad), before she could go on a diet. Can you believe it? Here she is craving to lose weight, while totally incapable of seeing the irrationality of her ways. Please! Don't be like her or the others who continue to put off doing what must be done. Don't even put it off until tomorrow ("It'll be easier to get started first thing in the morning."); start right this minute.

If it's 9:00 am, 11:00 am, 3:00 pm, or whatever; start **now**! When it's time for your next meal, make it a meal that I've outlined in the seven daily menus. Don't sit around thinking of all the reasons you should put it off while you continue in your unhappy, overweight condition.

If you start right this moment, tomorrow will bring the loss of at least a few pounds; an excellent way to start the day.

How to Have Fun Getting There

Too many people approach the act of losing weight like zombies. They follow the recommendations and do what must be done, but never enjoy themselves. There is no reason to look forward to the next few weeks with trepidation. Losing weight can be just as much fun as you thought you were having when you put those extra pounds on.

I have watched dozens of overweight patients actually

become depressed *before* they even started to diet. They already felt that they were denying themselves, even before the fact. A week or more of this kind of attitude, and these individuals thought they could never again be happy.

Believe me, there is no reason to feel cheated or depressed while you are losing weight. Plan ahead. Think about your new slender figure, about the new clothes, and about the renewed vitality you'll have once you lose those excess pounds.

There is a section in the New Testament which explains (and I paraphrase loosely) that if a man making a sacrifice exhibits his discomfiture for others to see, he will not receive any reward in heaven. He will have already obtained his reward through the approval or sympathy that is given him on earth.

Think about that for a moment. I'm sure you will be able to see the similarity between the Bible's admonition, and the failure of many to lose weight.

If you are going to walk around with a "sour-puss," looking dejected and put-upon, you will probably get the sympathy (but not the understanding) of those around you.

That may be the only thing you get, however. Subconsciously, you may accept the sympathy as a reward for your dieting efforts. If so, you probably will not obtain the reward of lasting slenderness. Face it! You will have already been given your reward (the sympathy of others); you don't deserve anything additional in your mind.

What I have been stressing here is your need to be "**UP.**" Don't approach your weight loss program as something that is distasteful. Look at it as a new experience, a new adventure that will not only be exciting, but will also bring you the greatest reward—self-respect. As you begin to lose those extra pounds, look forward to both your emotional and physical rewards. Let no one know that you are dieting, and your reward will be slenderness.

Why Stanley F. Wanted to Be Sensual

Stanley wasn't excessively heavy. When he first sought help with his weight, he only needed to lose 22 pounds.

During the time that he came to me, I learned that his wife had left him, and had taken their 18-month-old son with her. She had gone back to New Jersey, and her departing remark was, "I never want to see you or Florida again."

It isn't too difficult to understand Stanley's feelings of inferiority and depression. Perhaps you have had a similar tragedy in your own life.

In any event, Stanley wanted to lose weight because he felt this would make him attractive to women. Stanley honestly wanted to be sensual, hoping that this alone would make his wife see the "error of her ways."

During the four weeks that Stanley came to my office, we became well-acquainted. I learned that he lacked confidence, didn't like mirrors (because of what they reflected), and that he wanted to attract women.

During the last part of the second week on the program, though, there seemed to be a change in Stanley's attitude. He seemed to be in better spirits.

When the opportunity arose, I questioned him about this. He told me that when he first started on the Super 500 Program, his only concern was to make others like him. Now, however, he felt that whether or not others liked him, he would like himself. He was not going to lose weight for someone else; he was going to do it for himself!

He further related that before he began to lose weight, he was quite impressed by other men: men who had nice cars, beautiful clothes, and good physiques. Now, after only two weeks, he felt that although he still liked these material things, it was more important to like himself. He was not going to lose weight or otherwise change himself, unless he felt it would make *him* better, inside.

I realize that this story may appear long, and perhaps is not even strictly related to the loss of weight, but I feel that Stanley (who, by the way, did lose the 22 pounds) is an excellent example of so many other patients who initially attempted to lose weight for "someone else."

Incidentally, Stanley no longer lives in Florida. He has returned to New Jersey, and from what I understand, he and his wife are giving it another try. Apparently she didn't mean what she said about not ever wanting to see him again.

Unfortunately though, what she said about not wanting to see Florida seems to have been true.

Why You Will Enjoy the Super 500 Program

In a previous paragraph I stated that you should enjoy losing weight. I'll bet you've never heard anyone say that before. The fact is that everyone who follows the Super 500 Program as directed will actually enjoy themselves. That's Right! *Enjoy Themselves.*

There is absolutely no reason to dread the next few weeks. The Super 500 is so easy to follow, and is so successful in melting those unwanted pounds away, that you will honestly feel as if you've been partying, when all the time you've been "dieting."

If you follow the directions exactly, you will never have a chance to get bored. Before you realize you're controlling your weight, you will have lost a dozen pounds or more, and will already be on the interim program. The dieting portion of the program will be over before you get used to it. The one-week interim period, with all the wonderful food and drink it offers, will seem like a New Year's Eve party. How could you possibly fail to have a good time losing weight?

Don't forget: follow the directions exactly. Eat everything that is permitted, take the few minutes necessary to prepare those scrumptious satisfiers, and discard any excess quantities of food that should not be eaten (Stop trying to be a human garbage-disposal. Whether or not you finish everything in sight, there will still be people in the world who must go hungry. Stop feeling that it's a sin to waste food).

If you will do this, the people around you will think you are trying to "put on a few pounds," while all the time excess weight will be literally melting from your body. What a way to "diet."

How Joyce C. Did It with "Gusto"

Joyce was 17 years old when she first came to see me. At 5'2" and carrying 139 pounds, she certainly didn't look like the vivacious person I came to know. I must admit that when I first saw Joyce she was fairly attractive. Her facial features and the way she fixed her hair and applied make-up did her justice. Unfortunately, those extra pounds she was carrying didn't help her looks.

From the very first day of her program, Joyce exuded a certain cheerfulness. With each pound that was dropped by the wayside, she became more excited and happy. She virtually "bounced" through the twenty-one-day program, and by the end of the seven-day interim period, Joyce had achieved her goal.

Eighteen pounds had been lost, and now, at 121 pounds, she was beautiful. As an added reward for her perseverance, Joyce's mother took her shopping for a complete, new wardrobe. I doubt that I have ever seen any young woman more jubilant or bubbling over with new-found awareness of herself.

When I spoke with Joyce after she had achieved her weight loss goals, I asked her why she was so "bouncy," so "up." She told me that when she first began the program, she promised herself she wouldn't allow anything to "get the best of her." She had to force herself to act cheerful that very first day, but the next morning when she saw that she had already dropped two pounds, she *was* cheerful.

From that point on, she honestly did feel great. She remained excited throughout the program, and was ecstatic when, in less than a month, she had achieved her goal.

Joyce did it with "gusto." She innately knew what so many other dieters must learn: "As you think, so shall ye be."

I hope that relating this story of how one young woman mentally prepared herself for weight reduction, will motivate you to do the same. As I have said before: you can truly enjoy losing weight when you follow the *Super 500 Rapid Weight Loss Program.*

CHAPTER 7

HOW YOU BENEFIT
FROM THE SUPER 500 EXPANSION

Every weight loss program I have ever seen in the past has been both tedious and restrictive. Until the Super 500 Program, losing weight required enormous willpower. Although a number of overweight people have succeeded in slimming down even when faced with these boring "diets," I can't see why anyone would want to be denied good food unnecessarily.

When the Super 500 Program was first being formulated, it contained a number of restrictive measures. Fortunately, many patients took the time and effort to constructively criticize the diet. They further pointed out that although the basic concept was excellent, the program contained a number of faults, of which I was unaware. Each time a new idea was incorporated into the weight loss plan, the program became both easier and more enticing to a larger number of people. One patient, Sharon B., was so adamant in her feelings, that the incorporation of the satisfiers resulted primarily from her proddings.

Sharon and the Slenderizing Thickshake

I don't think Sharon was ever more than 10 or 15 pounds overweight in her life. She was very conscious of her figure, and time and again had lost those excess pounds, only to regain them one more time. Truthfully, when Sharon first came to see me, she was more interested in maintaining her weight than in losing a few pounds. She knew that she could lose the excess weight, but didn't know how to keep it off without continuous dieting.

Since the original Super 500 Program contained a weight-maintenance plan, Sharon felt she could benefit from it. Once she had lost the eight extra pounds she was carrying, she was put on this maintenance portion of the program: three weeks later she was back.

"This maintenance procedure seems to work, but I think something has to be done to make it more enjoyable," she complained.

"What do you mean?" I asked.

"Well, to tell you the truth" she started, "the between-meal snacks are *BORING*. There just isn't enough variety in them, and most don't satisfy my craving for something sweet. There must be a way you can include some enjoyable snacks without causing a weight gain."

I told Sharon to make a list of "forbidden" foods: sweets, desserts, and all the things she really enjoyed.

"You go home," I told her, "and draw up a list of all those foods you'd really like to see included in the maintenance program. Don't worry that they might contain too many calories. Just make the list and bring it back to me."

Three days later Sharon returned. Her list contained twelve different foods: foods that were excessively high in calories.

"I don't know what I can do to bring some of these foods into the maintenance program," I told her, "but let me give it a try."

That evening I spent many hours trying to alter the maintenance procedure to include at least one or two of the foods on Sharon's list. As I lay in bed tossing and turning, I realized that I had a craving for something sweet. Sharon's list of foods kept returning to my mind.

Finally, I got up and went to the kitchen.

"What can I make for myself?" I wondered. Suddenly, I realized that what I really had a craving for was a thick shake. I opened the freezer door and was reaching for the ice cream when it came to me.

"This must be what Sharon was talking about. She and all my other patients must go through this routine almost every day. No wonder they feel dissatisfied with the maintenance program."

I forced myself to put the ice cream back, but I didn't go back to bed. Instead, I sat at the kitchen table and pondered the problem of not being able to satisfy that craving inside me. After almost two hours, the solution came to mind.

I got up and prepared the first satisfier: the Creamy Banana Thick Shake. It took several tries before I got it just right, and I have since made several changes in the recipe (see Day Three Mid-Morning Satisfier), but there was no question about it; the craving for sweet, delicious snacks could be satisfied.

I spent the rest of the night and early morning designing additional satisfiers. When I finally got to my office, I had put together five delicious snacks; snacks that eaten in the right combination with other foods would not cause a regaining of weight. I was ecstatic!

Within three weeks, every maintenance program had been altered. A list of satisfiers was sent to every patient with directions for their preparation. Over the next few months, patients offerred suggestions and ideas. The list of satisfiers grew, and today there is virtually an unlimited number of sweet and satisfying snacks available that won't put the weight back on. I have included a number of these in the seven daily menus which appear in Chapter 5.

Now, as I look back on that night and the very first satisfier, I realize that Sharon was responsible for the inclusion of these wonderful, scrumptious desserts in the Super 500 Program.

Her list of "forbidden" foods was the stimulus that led me to formulate the satisfiers. Thank goodness she had put "A frosty thick shake" as her first choice, because it remained in my mind and I soon craved it. Had she reversed the order of her list and put her third choice (French Fries) first, I might never have come up with a solution to the problem of "forbidden" foods.

How Enjoying Yourself While Losing Weight Brings Greater Rewards

Have you ever begun a project, only to learn that after several days of devoted effort you were dissatisfied with the results? At that point you probably put the project aside.

"I'll do it another time," you may have told yourself. Today that project is probably still unfinished, gathering dust in some dark hiding place.

I have found that many individuals react in a similar manner when faced with a distasteful or tedious chore. In the past, weight reduction probably fell into this category. If you were not enjoying the particular dietary program you were following, or losing sufficient quantities of weight, you probably put the program aside. That is why enjoying yourself on a diet is so important.

As you proceed to lose weight on the Super 500 Program, you will find that you are enjoying what you are doing: the pounds are coming off, you feel energetic, and the foods you eat are delicious and satisfying. There is no reason to cast the program aside ... you are honestly having a good time.

As long as this remains true, as long as you do not feel denied or unhappy, you will continue with the program and continue melting those pounds away. The "greater rewards" you receive will be in the form of additional weight loss. You will, for once in your life, be able to get down to the weight which best suits you. You will not fall by the wayside, as has probably happened before. You will achieve your goals and remain slender for life. What better reward could be offered? What more could you expect from a weight-reduction program? Read on!

The Best Part: Realizing Your Dreams

In the very first chapter of this book, I made mention of the fact that most overweight people fantasize about what their lives would be like if they could lose their excess weight. Romance, love, success, a better job, new awareness of yourself, and increased self-respect are only some of the recurring fantasies.

Be assured though; these fantasies, these dreams, do come to pass. Time and time again I have seen previously overweight people, once they achieved slenderness, go out and make their dreams come true. The loss of a few pounds apparently has the ability to alter one's consciousness. People who have lost weight gain confidence. They are more sure of themselves, and no longer shy away from new experiences.

During the time these poeple were overweight, many of them shunned new relationships, refused to make new friends, didn't try to find a more satisfying job or attempt to better themselves.

Once they lost those unwanted pounds, however, they were no longer afraid of being rejected. They went forward and actively searched for a more fulfilling life. In most cases they were successful.

You too can look forward to being able to realize your dreams. Whatever those dreams are, you *will* be able to make them come true once you gain the self-confidence with which to strive for them. Once you begin to see yourself as the slender, attractive person you really are, the possibilities for a more satisfying life will open up before you: *that* is the best part of being slender.

How Linda Learned to Live

When she first came in to see me, Linda was thirty-five years old and more than 35 pounds overweight. Working as a billing clerk at a lumber yard, she was stuck off in a back room all day and never had the opportunity to meet the dozens of men who came in to buy building supplies. She had grown bitter and let herself go. She had little interest in what life had to offer, and if it weren't for her mother's constant prodding, she probably would never have come to see me at all.

Her weight loss was unremarkable; in six weeks she had reduced to 109 pounds, a perfect weight for her 5'3" height.

The change that was made in her personality, however, *was* remarkable. In all the years I have treated the problem of obesity, I have never seen such a total alteration in a person's appearance and attitude.

Within seven months of achieving her weight-loss goals, Linda's life style had changed dramatically. I spoke with her mother recently, and found out that Linda was now selling real estate. Once she had slimmed down, she had gone to school at night, had taken her real estate test, and had passed with flying colors.

She was making good money and had moved from the duplex in which she had been living. She now owned an oceanfront condominium, had met a man she really liked, was playing raquetball several times a week, and was generally "enjoying the heck out of life." I was stunned! If you had met Linda when she first came to my office, you would understand why. The changes that had been made in her life by the loss of that excess weight were incredible. Yet they had occurred.

If someone like Linda could become a warm and loving person, if someone like Linda could become successful in both her career and her personal life, I believe *everyone* can realize their dreams once they see themselves as slender, attractive individuals.

The Extra Benefit—Holding Your Own

As I mentioned in a previous section, the Super 500 Program incorporates a maintenace plan. Once you have achieved slenderness, you do not want to have to do it over again. By following the recommendations I have made in the final chapter of this book, you will have no problem maintaining your new weight—forever!

There isn't another dietary program anywhere that can make this statement, to my knowledge. Of course, if you continue to diet and restrict the intake of the foods you enjoy, you can stay thin. But to be able to eat out at restaurants, attend festive occasions, and generally have a ball when it comes to "eats and drinks" was unheard of before the Super 500 Maintenance Program.

Once you are slender, you will understand more fully why this extra benefit of the *Super 500 Rapid Weight Loss Program* is so exciting.

CHAPTER 8

HOW TO USE THE INTERIM PROGRAM FOR TOTAL SLENDERNESS

Once you have completed your twenty-one day, rapid weight loss program, you should (as I mentioned earlier), proceed to the interim program. By following the instructions outlined in this chapter, you will have no problem losing an additional two to five pounds.

For one week, you will eat normally, without excessive restrictions or the need to pay an inordinate amount of attention to your intake. At the end of this seven-day interim period, you may either proceed to the maintenance program which I mentioned in the previous chapter (see Chapter 7 for complete, detailed instructions on how to proceed), or you may still require the loss of additional weight. If you must lose more weight, you should return to Chapter 5 and begin a second, twenty-one day, rapid weight-loss program. Proceed as you did originally, using the seven daily menus to assist you in choosing the foods to eat. At the end of the second twenty-one days, you should again return to this chapter and the interim program.

Continue in this fashion until you have attained your desired weight. At that point, proceed to Chapter 7 for the maintenance program which best suits you.

How You Can Begin Eating Three Satisfying Meals Each Day

Were you aware that most obese individuals rarely eat three meals daily? It's true! Based on my records, fewer than 7 percent of my overweight patients reported that they ate three regular meals. When this fact first became evident, I attempted to find the reason for it. Although I interviewed a great number of overweight individuals, I was unable to find a specific cause.

However, I did find a generalized trait that existed in all these individuals; a trait which I feel is primarily responsible for this habit of not eating three regular meals daily. This trait, to put it simply, is *spontaneity*.

My interviews revealed that each and every obese individual exhibited this trait. To these individuals, living is more or less a spontaneous event: the less regimentation the better. Because of this, many of them eat wherever and whenever they get the urge. They dislike being "forced" to eat their meals at predetermined times.

Certainly, many of them are required to eat according to some imposed schedule (i.e., school and work lunch times, home-cooked meals at specific hours, etc.), but that isn't to say they like it. If they were allowed to eat in accordance with their own wishes, these individuals would find themselves eating at all times of the day and night.

Unfortunately, society restricts and prevents this spontaneity from being exhibited in most cases. Since there are prescribed times for breakfast, lunch and dinner, society generally "forces" most of us to eat according to a dictated schedule.

Think about this for a minute; forget, for the moment, what other (skinny) people do. Isn't it true that you, on occasion, have a craving for something to eat or drink between meals? Don't you find yourself sometimes wishing it were time for lunch or dinner long before the scheduled meal? If you are like most people, I am sure you have had this experience. Let's examine what it means.

You, as an individual, would like to eat and drink at odd times and whenever you have the desire to do so. But because your life is ruled by clocks and routine, you are forced to put off eating even though you feel hungry. Then, when the clock or routine permits, you probably find yourself overeating.

Not very mysterious, is it? You are prevented from eating when you are hungry, so your body craves more food when it is "time" to eat. If you were able to act spontaneously and eat whenever you felt like it, you would probably never have become overweight in the first place. Now, however, when you eat spontaneously, you probably find yourself also being "forced" to eat the next scheduled meal, even though you're not hungry. I have seen this happen more times than I care to remember.

For example, a man or woman feels a certain craving for something to eat while at work. It is 3:00 pm, and although he had lunch at the usual time, he still feels a little hungry. Perhaps he finds a candy machine, or the afternoon coffee break gives him an opportunity to get a piece of cake. In any event, for the purpose of this story, let us assume that he does satisfy his desire for a snack.

On returning home in the evening, he finds that his wife has dinner waiting as usual. To avoid offending her, this man will probably sit down to dinner and proceed to eat a full meal. Sometimes he may even eat *more* than usual because he subconsciously feels guilty about not really being hungry. The mental machinations may go something like this:

"She always prepares a fine meal for me, and I foolishly ruined my appetite by eating that snack this afternoon. I certainly don't want her to think that I don't appreciate the food she prepares, so I guess I'll take another serving." Or, "I wouldn't want her to feel that I think so little of her time that I'd go out and eat junk, all the time knowing she'd have a full meal ready when I got home." Or, "I best not say anything about not being hungry. I don't want to hurt her feelings."

I wish I could report that the above example is in some way unusual, but it isn't. If you are prevented from eating when you truly desire food, you will probably overstuff yourself at the earliest opportunity; if you do satisfy your craving for food at a time that doesn't coincide with your daily schedule, you'll probably find yourself eating as much, if not more, than you should at the next meal.

No matter what you do about your craving for food, if that craving is out of sync with your daily schedule, you'll probably find yourself gaining weight as a result of your spontaneous nature. Unless you can restructure your life style and eat only when you are hungry, you will pay the price for your spontaneity, and that price will be obesity.

Getting back to the fact that most obese people don't eat three meals a day, I would like to illustrate the most probable reason for this. Remember, however, that your spontaneous nature is the true, underlying motivation for what you do.

Whether, as in the above example, you satisfy your craving for a mid-afternoon snack or you deny your craving, the fact is that you will probably overeat at dinner time.

These large evening meals (and/or late night snacking) are the real reason most overweight people don't eat three meals a day. The food contained in these meals is rarely digested completely before the person retires for the evening. Because of this, the food (which is still in the stomach and upper digestive tract) is slowly digested during sleep.

Since you are not performing any calorie-burning activities while sleeping, the body doesn't require these extra calories that are being pumped into the blood stream. In an effort to conserve energy, however, the body refuses to let these calories be wasted. Instead, the miraculous physiology of the body acts to store them for future needs.

And how does the body do this? As fat, that's how! Each calorie that isn't immediately needed for energy expenditure ultimately becomes a fat molecule, which is then stored in the form of fat reserves throughout your body. Additionally, since your body digests these late evening meals and snacks more slowly because of your inactivity, there will still be a high concentration of sugar in your bloodstream when you first awaken in the morning.

For this reason, many overweight people don't eat breakfast upon arising. Several hours later, though, they are literally starving to death. The activity of getting up, getting dressed and moving about reduces the blood sugar level and stimulates the appetite. Another day begins with a craving for food that is out of sync with the daily schedule.

Simply put, the fact that you are probably of a spontaneous nature is the reason you eat at odd times, and out of order with your daily routine. This, as I've said before, often results in eating overly large evening meals or late night snacks. In turn, this produces increased blood sugar levels upon arising, which prevents any true desire for food the first thing in the morning. This means that you will once again have cravings for food and drink at times that are not set aside for these activities. The vicious cycle continues!

The Miracle of the Midday Meal

If you can see yourself in the above example, you may want to try something that has been proven beneficial over the years: a large midday meal.

Most Americans eat their biggest meal in the evening. If you are one of these people, you should attempt to alter your dietary intake sufficiently to permit you to eat dinner (your largest meal) at noon. You will then be having your largest meal at midday instead of in the evening.

Let's see what this would do. First, because you are eating quite a bit at lunch time, you won't have any midafternoon cravings. Second, as long as you don't overdo it or gorge yourself, you will have an adequate blood sugar level during the late afternoon without the unwanted side effect of feeling drowsy. While others around you may be slowing down and feeling the afternoon slump, you will be energetic and full of "spunk." Third, you will be eating a light dinner, and will therefore not overburden the digestive tract late at night. As a result there will be no excess food remaining in the stomach when you retire for the evening, and your blood sugar levels will be normal. You should have no trouble getting to sleep.

When you awaken the next morning you will be ready for breakfast, although you may initially require a stimulant to get the digestive juices flowing. This is because after several years of not eating breakfast, the body becomes accustomed to this fact and doesn't produce the necessary digestive chemicals early in the morning. This problem will take care of itself once you form the new habit of eating breakfast every day.

The simple act of eating breakfast will allay any desire for food until lunch time. If you should note a craving for food prior to lunch, however, a small snack, a satisfier, should suffice, which should not interfere with your lunch time appetite. By continuing in this fashion, you will instill the habit of eating your largest meal at the noon hour.

Miraculously, because you are still active during the late afternoon, the body will not permit the excess calories you consume to be deposited as fat. Instead, the increased sugar level in the blood will act as an energy reserve for the things you must still accomplish before your evening meal. Instead of being stored in the form of fat, the calories will now be used to produce energy. You will now be burning off those excess calories instead of storing them.

By the simple habit of eating your biggest meal at noon time, you will have prevented the most common cause of obesity: eating spontaneously, and out of sync with your daily routine.

Snacks Need Not Be a Problem

While reading the previous paragraphs, you may have gotten the impression that between-meal snacks were a "no-no." This, however, is not true. Between-meal snacks are fine, so long as you eat them judiciously. Don't overdo it!

The satisfiers I have included in the seven daily menus can be taken at just about any time. A piece of fruit, a raw vegetable or a vegetable juice cocktail all make good between-meal snacks. Four satisfiers, six pieces of fruit or a bushel of raw vegetables are not the answer though. You must be judicious!

The real reason you crave food between meals is that your blood sugar level has been lowered. This activates your appetite, and you subconsciously try to raise your blood sugar level by eating something.

That is why so many people crave sweets at these times—they represent an easily digested form of sugar. If you keep this fact in mind, you will always remember that what you are trying to do is raise your blood sugar levels: not stave off the spectre of "death by starvation."

Because it takes time for the sugar level of the blood to rise, many overweight people eat inordinate amounts of food before feeling satisfied. Then, a half-hour later, they realize they are "stuffed." If they would only take a small amount of food, then wait several minutes, they would find that their cravings have been satisfied. All they have to do is give their bodies a chance to absorb the food they've eaten and to increase their blood sugar levels. Unfortunately, many obese individuals overeat long before their bodies have an opportunity to signal that they are satisfied. The excess calories that continue to be absorbed over the next several hours are then stored as fat. The body has no way of using up the excess energy (calories) being pumped into the bloodstream.

So, although there is no reason to deny yourself a snack when you desire one, you must use common sense and not overdo it. A simple method I have found that works for just about everyone, is to prepare snacks long before you crave them. When you first get up in the morning, you may want to put aside a reasonable quantity of food that you will be eating as snacks: perhaps a piece of fruit before lunch and some raw carrot sticks prior to your evening meal. By doing this and promising yourself that you will not eat anything else, you will be able to increase your blood sugar levels as needed without increasing your weight. You'll be surprised how a single piece of fruit can take away the jitters and the weakness that often accompanies lowered blood sugar levels. Just give it a chance to be absorbed.

How to Choose the Interim Program You'll Like Best

Keeping in mind my previous statements about spontaneity and judiciousness when eating, it is now time to formulate an interim program for yourself that you will enjoy. Don't forget that during this one week period, we still want to reduce your weight by at least two pounds, preferably five. At the same time, however, we want to be assured of enjoying the intermission. Consequently, there are a few rules which must be followed. If you will but incorporate these rules into your daily routine, you will never have a problem with obesity again. But for now, these rules must be used to produce both an enjoyable interim program and the loss of an additional two to five pounds.

Rules to Follow to Make Your Interim Program Enjoyable

1) Every morning drink at least an eight to twelve ounce glass of Sparkling Lemon Tonic. (See Day Three Breakfast Menu for directions on preparation.) This rule cannot be ignored; it is essential, and following it produces two results: A) your digestive system will be stimulated to produce the necessary chemicals required for the digestion of early morning food; B) by drinking the Tonic at least fifteen minutes before eating any food, you will have initiated the appropriate body responses (i.e. a feeling of fullness prior to food intake).

2) Always eat your three meals at regular intervals. Do not permit yourself to eat spontaneously and injudiciously.

3) Between meal snacks are permitted, but follow the rules. Follow the recommendations I've made in the previous section and you'll have no problem.

4) Adjust your daily routine to make your midday meal the biggest one of the day. At the evening meal, have soup and a salad, a sandwich or some other relatively light fare. You'll be surprised how important this simple adjustment will be in maintaining your lowered weight later on.

That's really all there is to it. You don't have to be overly strict with yourself. Just try to use your head when you are going to eat, and your body will take care of the rest. If you crave something sweet, take a satisfier. If you really are hungry, supplement your meals with a low calorie filler like salad, or unbuttered vegetables. But, as I've said before, don't be too serious. You deserve to enjoy yourself during this interim period. Prepare your snacks before hand; give your body a chance to "tell" you that it's satisfied before you gorge yourself. Eating slowly is perhaps the best way to accomplish this. But, by all means, eat the foods you normally enjoy. For the moment, at least, forget about calories. This is your one-week vacation from dieting—**ENJOY.**

Food For Thought

If you, like many of my patients, are concerned that you will "blow the whole thing" during this one-week interim period, you may gain confidence from the following recommended foods. Just remember, if you'd rather, you may eat all the foods you enjoy, as long as you're careful about the quantities you consume.

Breakfasts that Get the Day Started Right

Keeping in mind the rules you must follow during this one-week interim period, you may find the following breakfast suggestions exceptionally satisfying.

Cereals: You may eat any and all cereal breakfast foods. Remember: one cup of dry, flaked or puffed cereal or ¾ cup of cooked cereal is an adequate serving. Give your body the opportunity to let you know it is satisfied with that amount. Don't eat a giant portion out of habit.

Eggs: Almost everyone enjoys eggs for breakfast. Prepare them any way you like (Eggs Benedict?) but eat just one. I know that you probably are used to eating two, but you'll soon learn that one egg is just as filling and satisfying. Order or cook just one, with a single slice of buttered toast. I guarantee that you won't know the difference between eating one or two eggs half an hour after you've finished.

Other Foods: You may have a special food you enjoy for breakfast. Don't worry about the calories it contains. If you enjoy it, eat it. The only caution is: don't overdo it. Keep the portions down in size, and you'll have no problem losing those extra pounds.

Sandwiches that Satisfy

I for one, am especially fond of sandwiches. However, the major problem with them, from a weight standpoint, is the number of calories they contain. One way to keep the calories down while keeping the enjoyment up is as follows: freeze a loaf of your favorite bread; when it is frozen, use a serrated knife to cut a single slice into two. Voila! You now have two slices of bread for your sandwich, and the calories have instantly been cut in half.

When making your sandwiches, don't be too conservative. Use all the garnishes at your disposal, such as lettuce, tomato, onion, and all the herbs and spices you find appealing. If you like butter or mayo on your sandwich, go ahead and use it. Just don't overdo it!

One combination that I truly enjoy is a sandwich (almost any kind of luncheon meat or cheese can be used) piled high with the following:

¼ head of lettuce, shredded

½ unpeeled cucumber, chopped

½ tomato, chopped

1 stalk celery, diced fine

½ cup apple cider vinegar

Toss all the ingredients together, then add ¼ tsp. each of oregano, chopped parsley, and thyme. Let the mixture set in the refrigerator for at least two hours. When ready to serve, spoon a large quantity of this salad mix (well drained) over your favorite meat and cheese sandwich. Spread a large amount of "spicy brown" mustard on the top slice (actually a half slice) of bread. A taste treat to be sure!

If you have some favorite sandwich that you really enjoy, this is the time to have it. By reducing the quantity of the various sandwich fillers, and using the trick of only a single slice of bread to make the sandwich, you'll have no trouble with your weight loss.

Lunches You'll Look Forward To

As I mentioned in a previous section, your midday meal should be your largest meal. If you follow this recommendation, you will be pleasantly surprised at the results. Never again will you have to concern yourself with obesity; never again will you worry about your weight. Simply eat dinner at lunchtime, and you will be on your way to permanent slenderness. During this one-week interim period, I would suggest that you eat for lunch whatever you normally have for dinner.

Prior to starting on the Super 500 Program, I am sure you had a fairly predictable dinner schedule. At this time, there is no reason to alter your food intake. If, for instance, you enjoy pizza (or pasta, or potatoes, etc.), feel free to enjoy these foods during this week. Instead of having them at dinner time, however, eat them at your midday meal. By all means, don't overdo it.

If you eat the foods you enjoy, you will have little craving or desire to eat excessively. You will not feel "denied," and therefore self-pity will not lead you to indiscretion. Even if the foods you usually ate before the Super 500 Program were high in calories, don't be overly concerned. The interim period was designed to be enjoyed. Eat what you like, but not as much as you normally would, and you will still lose an additional few pounds without sacrifice. When you know you'll be eating what you enjoy, you will definitely look forward to lunch.

How to Create Scrumptious Salads

I must admit that most dieters consider salads to be "rabbit food." In the past, every time they wanted to lose a few pounds, they were advised to eat raw vegetables or salads. I have been told by patients however, that most of the time these salads consisted of nothing more than lettuce, tomato, oil and vinegar. Certainly these ingredients often form the basis of a good salad; but by themselves, they can be very dull. If you will take the opportunity during this one-week interim period to experiment, I think you will find that raw vegetables and salads can be both nutritious and delicious.

Try some of the following suggestions, and I think you'll be both surprised and pleased at how good salads can be.

"Never at the Waldorf" Salad

Combine 3 cups of crisp, shredded cabbage with an 8 oz. can (1 cup drained) of low-calorie pineapple tidbits. Toss with 1 cup of diced apple and ½ cup of chopped celery. Add ½ cup of low-calorie mayonnaise and mix until coated. Makes 6 scrumptious salad servings.

Stuffed Tomatoes

Put the contents of a 9 oz. package of Italian green beans, cooked according to directions and drained, in a large bowl. Add a 3 oz. jar of drained, sliced mushrooms, 2 tbs. Italian salad dressing, ¼ cup of chopped scallions (green onions) and season with salt and freshly ground pepper to taste. Toss and refrigerate.

While this stuffing mixture is being chilled, cut off the tops of 6 medium sized, ripe tomatoes and scoop out the centers with a spoon. Place them upside down on a paper towel to drain. Sprinkle the insides of the tomatoes with salt, fill with the stuffing mixture, then serve. This recipe is so low in calories that you can eat as many of the stuffed tomatoes as you want. The only precaution I would offer is not to stuff yourself. You must keep in mind my advice regarding the amount of food you used to eat in the past. It is unnecessary to gorge yourself. Eat one tomato, and if you are still hungry after 15 minutes, have another. Give your body a chance to tell you it is satisfied.

Curried Shrimp

Drain two 4 oz. cans (1 cup) of shrimp. Mix with 2 tbs. of fresh lemon juice, 1 cup of finely chopped celery and 2 tbs. of freshly snipped parsley. Add ½ cup of low-calorie mayonnaise to which ½ tsp. of curry powder has been added. Toss gently with 4 cups of lettuce torn into bite-sized pieces. Garnish with 2 eggs that have been hard cooked and sliced. Season with salt and pepper to taste. Makes 6 servings.

Low-Calorie Tuna Salad

Mix ¾ cup of wine vinegar with 2 tsps. of sugar and 1½ tsps. of crushed, dried basil leaves. Chill in the regrigerator.

Toss 6 cups of torn lettuce with 2 cans of drained, flaked, water-packed tuna; 1½ cups of chopped fresh tomatoes; ½ a chopped onion, and ½ cup of sliced celery. Add the chilled dressing, toss gently and serve. Makes six scrumptious salads.

The four recipes above make use of fresh raw vegetables (except for the Italian green beans), and I am sure you can create any number of excellent variations on these basic themes. The secret, as always, is to be inventive; try new things. When creating, always try to use ingredients that contain the least amount of calories, but never settle for "dullness." For instance, the following chart indicates that there are certain seasonings that go well with different vegetables. Don't follow these recommendations blindly; instead, strive for flavors that stimulate your own palate.

Vegetable Seasonings

Concocting your own vegetable and salad combinations can be fun. Some of the basics of vegetable seasoning follow. Use what you think you'd enjoy, but don't be afraid to try new flavorings.

Vegetables usually have a delicate flavor and often require some additional spice to make them interesting. The following guide will be a "life-saver" when it comes to sprucing up those vegetable dishes. Try several combinations to determine which you like best, then be sure to record these recipes where you will come across them in the future. You will find that vegetables and salads can become an integral part of your every day menu, and you won't gain back those pounds that you've already lost.

Artichokes: **bay leaves, thyme**
Asparagus: **caraway seed, sesame seed, and tarragon**

Green Beans:	basil, bay leaves, dill, marjoram, oregano, savory
Lima Beans:	chili powder, curry, sage
Baked Beans:	cloves, ginger
Beets:	caraway seed, cloves, nutmeg, tarragon
Broccoli:	mustard, oregano
Brussels Sprouts:	caraway seed, nutmeg, sage
Cabbage:	allspice, basil, celery seed, nutmeg
Carrots:	bay leaves, chives, curry, dill, ginger, mace
Cauliflower:	caraway and celery seed, curry, dill
Corn:	chili powder, chives
Eggplant:	allspice, chili powder, sage, thyme
Mushrooms:	rosemary, tarragon
Onions:	basil, bay leaves, curry, ginger, mustard
Peas:	basil, chili powder, dill
Sweet Potatoes:	allspice, cardamon, cinnamon, nutmeg
White Potatoes:	basil, bay leaves, caraway and celery seed, sesame seed, chives, dill
Spinach:	allspice, cinnamon, dill, mace
Summer Squash:	basil, bay leaves, mace
Winter Squash:	allspice, cinnamon, cloves, ginger
Tomatoes:	basil, bay leaves, curry, dill, oregano, sage
Turnips:	allspice, dill, oregano

Salad Dressings that Stimulate the Palate

There is an old maxim that says, "Clothes make the man." It is no less true that dressings make the salad. Herewith are several dressings that are low in calories but high in flavor. Use them whenever you feel like having a basic lettuce and tomato salad. You will find that they do much to alter the flavor and enjoyment of your meals.

Saucey Salad Dressing

Dissolve 1¼ tsp. of unflavored gelatin in ½ cup of tomato juice. Bring to a boil over medium heat, and add 1½ tsp. dry salad dressing mix, 2 tbs. vinegar, and 1 additional cup of tomato juice. Stir well, remove from heat and chill. Makes a delicious and almost calorie-free dressing. Stir before using though as the seasonings sink to the bottom.

Tomato Dressing

Combine 1 cup of tomato sauce, 2 tbs. vinegar, 1 tsp. dried onion flakes, 1 tsp. Worcestershire sauce, and ½ tsp. each of salt, dillweed, and crushed, dried, basil leaves. Use an electric blender to mix well. Two tablespoons equal one serving.

Gourmet's "Delite"

This dressing is also very low in calories and may be used freely. Combine 1 tbs. cornstarch with ½ tsp. dry mustard and 1 cup of cold water. Heat until thickened, stirring constantly. Remove from heat and allow mixture to cool at room temperature.

Once the cornstarch mixture reaches room temperature, add ¼ cup each of vinegar and catsup, ½ tsp. each of paprika, prepared horseradish, Worcestershire sauce, and dried garlic flakes (not salt). Season with a dash of non-caloric liquid sweetener, and salt to taste. Chill and stir well before serving. Use freely.

Delectable Dinners Especially for You

As I mentioned earlier, dinner (supper) should not be your heaviest or largest meal. Since you will be eating sufficient amounts of food at lunch time, you do not need overly large evening meals. The best suggestion I can make regarding dinner is that you experiment. I have found that most patients are satisfied with one or more of the following items, as desired.

1) Soup, 2) Salad, 3) or a Sandwich

Try a steaming bowl of Manhattan-style clam chowder with your favorite sandwich, or a cool and scrumptious salad to which your favorite sandwich filling has been added. Melba toast on the side completes the makings of the sandwich.

In any event, don't allow yourself to maintain the preconceived thought that soup and a sandwich (or soup and a salad, etc.) will be insufficient to "fill you." If you eat slowly without being tense, you will find that you will do "very nicely, thank you."

By preventing yourself from overindulging at your evening meal, you will nurture a slenderizing habit that will serve you well in the future. Once again, though, I remind you to experiment. Try new and different foods; break the old habits of improper eating. You'll find that there are innumerable delicious foods you haven't tasted yet.

CHAPTER 9

HOW TO AVOID SETBACKS

Intermittent setbacks are perhaps the most frequent cause of failure during a diet. Although the Super 500 Program is designed to virtually eliminate the possibility of setback, there have been times in the past when patients reported that they fell by the wayside because of unforseen circumstances.

The increased stress that accompanies a mate's or child's illness, when job pressures grow, or when unanticipated events occur, can easily cause you to lose sight of your slenderness goal. After a day or two of not "paying attention to business," you find yourself regaining the pounds you have already lost. You may become depressed or anxious, and as a result, begin eating even more food than before.

This sequence of events is common. Generally, the involved dieters rationalize their failure to continue dieting in this way:

"How can I pay attention to a diet when I have to devote so much time and attention to my sick son?" In the above statement, you can replace "my sick son," with any or all of the following:

visiting relatives

entertaining prospective clients

preparing for the upcoming (anniversary, birthday, wedding)

getting ahead in a job

enjoying a vacation

As you can see, there are any number of rationalizations that people use to lessen the guilt feelings associated with going off their diets. All I can say is, *don't do it!* Don't allow yourself to give up on what you really want, and that is a slender body you can be proud of.

I realize that you may find yourself under increased pressure and stress while dieting. This, however, is no reason to lose sight of your goals. Once you recognize that you will achieve the desired results in only a few weeks, it will be easier for you to disregard the temptation to "cheat."

Perhaps the best advice I can give you regarding the elimination of setbacks is to consciously forbid yourself to dwell on your diet. Don't allow yourself to think about the "supposed" sacrifices you are making. Dieting, especially when utilizing the Super 500 Program, is not some indescribable hardship. By now you have realized how easy it is to lose all those unwanted pounds. Don't let misplaced and uncalled for self-pity destroy what you are achieving.

How Sally Lost Those Last Few Pounds

Although most people think of setbacks as occuring primarily during the initial phases of a dietary program, there is another kind of setback which must be avoided. I cautioned you earlier not to set your goals too low, and I suggested that you be honest with yourself when determining your true, ideal weight. Now, once you have committed yourself to losing those unnecessary pounds, you must be consciously aware of the need to achieve your goals. Don't allow yourself to experience the worst setback of all—not being totally and completely successful.

Sally had come to my office initially with a great desire to lose weight. She had only recently separated from her husband, and as many of us do, felt that losing weight was all she needed to get out of the "post-marital doldroms." It took a considerable amount of convincing to help Sally realize that she should lose weight for herself, not just for the anticipated psychological revenge she might get on her husband. Fortunately, Sally did come around. She could see that losing weight was more important to her own mental attitude than to her desire to somehow make her husband jealous. So for more than four weeks, Sally applied herself to becoming slender. Then (and I really don't know why), she and her husband resolved their differences and reconciled. At this point, Sally apparently lost all her motivation to lose the additional pounds. When she didn't keep one of her appointments, I had my nurse call her to see what was the matter. After some resistance, Sally agreed to come in to talk. When she arrived, we discussed her dietary program.

Sally, who had come to within seven pounds of her weight goal, was no longer motivated to lose the remaining weight. After more than 45 minutes, I finally persuaded her to attempt the loss of those last few pounds (Sally had originally been 33 pounds overweight).

Two weeks went by, but Sally continued to be seven pounds overweight. When I next saw her, she had rationalized that she really didn't need to lose any more weight.

"I'm fine," she told me. "I really don't feel fat, and I think my shape is super at my present weight. I don't want to lose any more."

"OK," I answered. "If you really feel totally pleased with yourself at this point, there is no reason for me to persuade you to lose those additional few pounds.

"If you are honestly proud of what you have accomplished, and don't feel that you are cheating yourself of the full pleasures of total success, you need not continue on with your weight loss program."

Sally explained that her husband thought she looked great. He didn't think she needed to lose any more weight and therefore she couldn't "psych" herself up. She rationalized her failure to continue on to achieve her goals.

After a few more minutes however, Sally admitted that she did feel a certain guilt about not pursuing her diet. She once again, albeit half-heartedly, promised to try to lose those last seven pounds. Yet one week later, there was still no reduction in weight.

"What's the matter?" I asked, when Sally returned to the office.

"I don't know. I just can't seen to stick to the program any longer."

"Don't worry" I replied, "if you are really serious about losing those last few pounds, I have the perfect solution to your problem.

"Are you sure you want to get rid of those pounds?" I asked.

"Yes" she responded, "now more than ever. Before I really wasn't certain, but now, after having tried unsuccessfully, I'll do just about anything to reach my goal."

"OK. This is what you have to do. Starting right this minute, you will go on a strict water fast for 48 hours. I guarantee that in less than two days you will have lost those last seven pounds. From this moment on, and for the next two days, you are to take no food or drink other than plain water. I know that this may sound a little severe, but I assure you, you will have no problems, and you will achieve your goal."

Needless to say, it took a while to convince Sally that a water fast was necessary. In the final analysis, though, she agreed to try it, and left my office with a positive attitude. Two days later Sally returned. Sure enough she had lost nine additional pounds and was ecstatic.

"I can't believe it," she bubbled. "The water fast wasn't even hard, and I lost those final pounds quicker than I could ever have imagined."

"I must admit that when I left the office last Tuesday, I promised myself that I would do exactly as you told me. Not because I thought it would work, but because I wanted to prove to you that I just couldn't lose those last few pounds. Today I feel great.

I'm sorry that I doubted you, but I just couldn't believe that the water fast would work so quickly. Thank you!"

For Sally, the loss of those last few pounds was more beneficial than losing the previous twenty-six. Not only had she reached her goal, but she had also kept faith with herself. Her confidence in being able to control her own body has, until this very day (almost two years after the event), resulted in a reawakening of her belief in her own personal worth.

Had she allowed herself the dubious luxury of not trying to lose those last few pounds, I doubt that she would have been able to maintain her new weight for very long. Sally is a perfect example of how important it is *not* to suffer the setback of not attaining what you are striving for.

Commitment Makes It Easy

You are probably wondering about the benefits of a water fast. You, too, probably think that going without food for a few days is a drastic and severe measure. I assure you, it is not.

If you seriously want to lose a few extra pounds, and you have already altered your eating habits by following the Super 500 Program for at least a few weeks, you will have no trouble on a water fast. The only individuals who have a problem with fasting are those who have been overindulging in food and drink. The excessive amount of toxic build-up in the bloodstream, which results from overindulging, often causes headaches and other symptoms when starting on a fast. However, if you have been eating sensibly for a few weeks, your body has had an opportunity to cleanse itself and balance the homeostatic mechanism.* You will have

---

* The homeostatic mechanism consists of all the physical, bio-chemical, and neurological (nerve) processes of the body. More specifically, those processes that are continually operating to maintain a balance among the various life-sustaining functions are known as the homeostatic processes.

(See Chapter 14, Body Temperature: Its Relationship to Weight Loss, for a specific example of how the homeostatic mechanism works to maintain proper body temperature.)

very little (if any) difficulty in following a water fast for a few days.

All you need do is stop eating! This may sound difficult, but once you try it, you'll find out how easy it really is. Don't be apprehensive. Don't listen to old wives tales about fasting. I repeat: just stop eating for a day or two. Drink nothing but plain water, and you will see yourself lose several pounds **overnight**.

If you commit yourself to trying a water fast, you will experience a decided increase in your own self-confidence. You will no longer be a slave to ritual. You will become increasingly aware of your body, and what it truly needs. In all seriousness, a short water fast is both helpful in weight reducing, and beneficial, and commitment makes it easy.

Answers to Your Questions

In a previous chapter, I mentioned that one of the reasons the *Super 500 Rapid Weight Loss Program* is so successful is because it incorporates a prescribed course of interpersonal communication between doctor and patient. Patients weren't left to their own devices. When they had problems or questions, there was always someone available that they could talk to. After several years of treating obesity through this revolutionary program, I came to the conclusion that almost every question that could be asked had been asked. I was therefore able to make up a question and answer sheet that included just about every important question and problem that had ever been brought up. At the present time, I find that patients rarely have questions that aren't answered on this sheet, and many patients go through the program completely without so much as a single question. I think this illustrates the benefit of having your mind put at ease, your questions answered, and your problems solved before they actually become problems.

The following is an exact duplicate of the question and answer sheet I give my patients. I am sure you will find it helpful.

Question:

Is it really necessary to have a complete physical examination just because I want to lose weight?

Answer:

Definitely! Although the great majority of overweight people I have seen in my office are in excellent health, I sometimes find a sub-clinical condition that will be adversely affected by altering the dietary intake. Many times, the present life style and eating habits effectively mask the underlying cause of certain symptoms.

A number of patients who believed their discomfort was due to obesity found that there was another, unrelated condition that was producing their symptoms. By all means, have both a complete physical examination and laboratory work-up before attempting to alter your weight. The few minutes it takes may well be repaid a thousand times over by the health information that it uncovers.

I do not wish to alarm you unnecessarily, but when it comes to your health, only a *complete* physical examination will serve to uncover any contraindicative conditions. By all means seek out your family physician and request an extensive examination.

Question:

I have had (such and such) surgery. Is it OK for me to go on a diet?

Answer:

Surgery, in and of itself, is rarely a contraindication to weight loss if you are overweight. At the same time, however, surgical intervention may produce an alteration in your homeostatic mechanism. Since I cannot ascertain exactly what surgical techniques may have been employed in your case, it is best that you contact the surgeon involved, and discuss your desire to lose weight with him.

It is extremely rare that weight reduction will become a contraindicated process due to a specific surgical procedure, but it is always best to consult with your surgeon and/or family physician before attempting any alteration in your life style. Take the time now to find out exactly where you stand health-wise, and you will most likely be able to proceed with your desired weight loss without any concerns.

Question:

I am currently taking ___medication for ___condition. My doctor has told me to continue taking this medication; can I still lose weight or will I have problems?

Answer:

Only the doctor who prescribes the medication can tell you the precise reason for taking it. It is also true that only a doctor who has treated you for a period of time (or who has access to your complete medical files) can accurately determine what you can and cannot do. Please contact the physician who prescribed the medication and ask him whether a restricted dietary regimen or loss of weight is permissible.

In all the years I have been helping people lose weight, I have yet to come across an individual whose intake of medicine was solely responsible for his not being able to diet. The Super 500 Program is completely balanced and nutritionally sound: you should have no problem obtaining your physician's approval to go ahead.

Question:

I am already following a prescribed diet. Can I still follow the Super 500 Program to lose weight?

Answer:

No! If your physician has ordered a specific diet for you, you should not alter your intake of food without his permission. If you are overweight, there is no reason why your doctor can't assist you in losing weight by modifying your current diet or altering the food intake permitted on the Super 500 Program to meet your specific needs. Do not proceed to lose weight or alter your life style without first consulting your personal physician.

Question:

Does the Super 500 Program work for everybody?

Answer:

Yes. If you are a normally healthy individual, there are no contraindications to proceeding with all phases of the *Super 500 Rapid Weight Loss Program*. If you suffer from some physical disorder, you can still utilize portions of the program without fear. (See Chapter 10 for a complete discussion of how to lose weight even if you have a health problem. The information contained in Chapter 10 may be especially important and beneficial for those of you who are on a prescribed diet already. I would therefore suggest that you bring Chapter 10 to the attention of your physician when you ask him about losing weight.)

Question:

What unusual symptoms or feelings might I experience while on the Super 500 Program?

Answer:

None. The Super 500 Program has been designed to produce nothing other than rapid weight loss. If you should find yourself experiencing some unusual symptoms while following the Super 500 Program, I suggest that you immediately consult your family physician. There is absolutely nothing contained in the program that should produce unwanted side effects or discomfort of any kind.

How to Ask Yourself the Really Big One

Most dieters have numerous questions, and I hope that the above answers will be as helpful to you as they have been to my patients. Before we get off the subject of questions, though, I would like to suggest that you spend a few minutes asking yourself the most important question of all:

"Do I really want to lose weight?"

You may think I am being facetious, but be assured that I am not. I have seen too many overweight patients who professed their desire to lose weight, then summarily disregarded all my suggestions.

If you are overweight and recognize that you are unhappy in your obesity, you may still need to search your conscience to decide whether you honestly want to lose those excess pounds. Because this book is primarily concerned with weight reduction, I do not feel that it is my place to delve into your subconscious mind to expose the underlying reasons why you may *not* want to lose weight.

I honestly feel that before you proceed to make a half-hearted attempt at weight loss, you should consider your motivations. If you are losing weight because someone else wants you to, if you are losing weight to please someone else, you may find that your results will be commensurate with, and indirectly proportional to, your feelings for that individual.

Without becoming overly repetitious, I would like to advise you to give some thought to what I have said. Before proceeding to your goals, decide in your mind once and for all whether and why you really want to lose weight.

If you do this *before* you begin your diet, you will find that no one and nothing can sway you from your goal. Once you have firmly established the course you wish to follow, you will be able to attain slenderness shortly. Once you realize that you want to lose weight for yourself and not for someone else, you will not feel threatened or disappointed by what others say and do as you start on the road to slenderness.

So long as you keep your own counsel, so long as you take pleasure in your own achievement, you will never have to take a back seat to anyone else's desires. Do it for **yourself.**

CHAPTER 10

HOW TO EAT YOUR WAY OUT OF OBESITY

On a number of occasions, I have been approached by overweight individuals who really needed to lose weight but just couldn't seem to get started. Although there were a variety of reasons why these individuals found themselves in this situation, a solution to their problem was necessary.

It took an enormous amount of trial and error, but a program that met the needs of these obese patients was finally formulated.

The Ultimate in Ease

After a number of attempts to get these reluctant, obese patients to lose weight, I finally came upon a method that has proven beneficial over the years.

It seems, that although these patients really and truly wanted to lose weight, they found themselves "cheating" after only a day or two on every diet they had ever tried.

When I first ran into this problem, I tried to motivate these individuals. I spent many hours trying to "psych them up" about the need to follow a prescribed diet. In essence, I tried to force them to lose weight.

It took quite a while for me to finally recognize and comprehend both their problems and my foolishness. These patients didn't need any "psyching up"; they were already motivated to lose their excess weight. They certainly couldn't be forced to lose weight; it had to be their own decision.

The major problem seemed to be their inability to follow a prescribed dietary program; one that recommended specific foods in specified quantities. When this thought finally hit me, I began to alter my approach to these patients' obesity problem.

Instead of trying to make them eat what I felt was important, I began to suggest that they continue eating what they enjoyed, but in smaller quantities. This may seem to be a simplistic approach to the obesity syndrome, but it works and it works well.

Of course if it was just as simple as all that, there wouldn't be an overweight person in the world. To admonish you to eat less is not the same as assisting you in the accomplishment of your goal. If you could simply decide that you weren't going to eat as much, you would surely be able to lose weight all by yourself. But it isn't as easy as all that.

To be successful, you must retrain yourself and alter your eating habits and patterns. Once you have accomplished this, you will find that obesity is no longer a problem. Once you have incorporated my suggestions into your life style, you will find that the pounds just seem to melt away. There will be no need to pay an inordinate amount of attention to your dietary intake; you'll be eating the foods you crave and enjoy.

Please don't expect overnight miracles, however. It will take some time for you to achieve your ideal weight. If you feel you must lose all your weight *rapidly*, I would suggest that you follow the twenty-one-day program as previously outlined. If, on the other hand, you recognize yourself as one of those individuals who always "cheats" on a diet, you may find the information contained in this chapter to be of particular benefit.

Since you will be eating the foods you enjoy, there will be little stress or pressure to cheat. After the first week of following this unique program, most of my suggestions will have become second nature. You won't have to consciously control your eating habits; they will have been altered to coincide with the attainment of slenderness.

By the end of the second week, you too will agree that this method of losing weight, although not very rapid, is very easy. If you follow the directions as outlined, you will find that the pounds continue to melt from your body.

Day in and day out, the fat will slowly disappear. You won't have to "try" to lose weight; the newly-formed eating habits you've learned, which will have become automatic, will take care of your obesity.

Although this method of weight reduction is easy, you must remember that the weight loss will be gradual. Don't expect more from this approach than it can deliver. Don't be overly concerned with whether or not you lose a pound or two on any particular day, because this program will work all by itself.

If you notice that you have gained a little because you overdid it the day before, don't worry. This is a normal consequence of overeating. The slender individual, as well as the obese one, will gain a pound and sometimes more, after eating an excessive quantity of food. The only difference is that the slender person rarely knows that his or her weight has gone up, because slender people don't weigh in every morning.

Several days after the episode which led to the weight gain, the slender person (and the obese person who is following this program) will have returned to his/her prior weight. The obese person, however, will continue to reduce. This program is designed to accomplish this without your ever being aware of it.

So, don't concern yourself or fret over the gain or loss of a few pounds. Know that if you continue to follow the program, if you instill the proper eating habits within your subconscious mind, you will eventually and inevitably reach your slenderness goal.

How to Lose Weight Even if You Do Have a Health Problem

Many overweight people who have a health problem seem to feel they are stuck with their obesity. They honestly believe that because they must take medication, limit their activities or otherwise restrict themselves, they will never again be slender. Don't believe it!

There is absolutely no reason why someone restricted in this way can't attain a desirable weight. If you are one of these individuals, you will find that by following the instructions in this chapter, you will become slender.

Before you attempt the loss of any weight, though, I again suggest that you consult with your personal physician. If he agrees that you would fare better and be healthier at a lesser weight and that you are presently eating properly, then you *will* be able to lose all those excess pounds easily and gradually by adhering to the following recommendations.

Let's face it: if your doctor feels that you are eating properly, the only possible cause of your obesity is that you are eating too much or at least more than is necessary at your present level of activity.

Even those individuals who suffer from hormonal irregularities can have their problem controlled by medication, and thus have their weight controlled by the simple expedient of reducing their intake of food.

In all modesty, I must confess that I am exceedingly proud of the unique approach to obesity in this chapter. Before I discovered this method of controlling weight, many patients were resigned to their obese condition. They had been told many times by other doctors that any kind of diet would be hazardous.

Now, because you will continue to obtain the proper nutrients and will not put undue or excessive stress on your physiological mechanisms, there is absolutely no reason you cannot attain a trim and slender figure.

So if you would like to lose those excess pounds but feel that a restrictive diet isn't for you, follow the suggestions in this chapter and be assured that you too will get thin.

Why Analyzing Your Food Intake Is Important

Are you aware that most overweight people don't realize what and how much food they eat? It's true! I am constantly amazed at the difference between what obese patients *think* they eat and what they actually consume.

Because most obese people are spontaneous in their eating habits, they rarely pay attention to what they eat. Only an accurate dietary analysis will expose the true variety and quantity of food they normally eat.

Don't take this suggestion lightly. If *you* think you are aware of everything you normally eat, then begin writing the foods and quantities down right now. In a short time, when you actually perform an accurate dietary analysis, you will be stunned by how much you forget.

To begin, get yourself three 8½" x 11" sheets of lined paper. Number the sheets 1, 2, and 3 at the top center of each page.

Each sheet will contain all the food eaten on three consecutive days. Immediately below each page number, print the word Item, move in two inches and print the word Quantity. Move to the right margin and print the word Symptom.

Next, on the top line of each sheet near the left hand margin, print the word Breakfast. Skip down about eight lines and print Mid-Morning Snacks. Skip another four to five lines and print Lunch or Dinner. Then skip to about five lines from the bottom of the page and print Afternoon Snacks. Now, turn the page over, and at the upper left-hand margin, print Dinner or Supper. Drop down twelve to fifteen lines and print Late Evening Snacks. At the bottom of the page, about five lines up, print the word Other.

Once you have done this on all three sheets of paper, you will be ready to begin your dietary analysis. You needn't wait until tomorrow, or some other day. Start right at this moment.

Don't rationalize that you'll put it off until after the party tomorrow night, or for some other equally faulty reason; do it *now*.

The following example illustrates what a typical dietary analysis would look like for one day.

Item	Quantity	Symptom
Breakfast		
Orange Juice	½ cup	
Eggs	2	
Butter, for frying	1 tbs.	
Salt	¼ tsp.	
Toast, white	2	
Coffee	2 cups	
Milk	¼ cup	
Sugar	2 heaping tsps.	
Mid-Morning Snacks		
Cookies	4	
Coffee	1	
Milk	⅛ cup	
Sugar	1 heaping tsp.	
Lunch (or Dinner)		
Hamburger	¼ lb.	headache starting
Bun	1	
French Fries	1 cup approximately	
Ketchup	1 tbs.	
Salt	¼ tsp.	
Soda	12 oz.	
Mid-Afternoon Snacks		
Candy Bar	1	headache gone
Chewing Gum	1 stick, sugarless	
Coffee	1 cup	
Milk	⅛ cup	
Sugar	1 heaping tsp.	

Dinner or Supper
Beer	2 cans (24 oz.)
Salad	1 cup
Salad Dressing	3 tbs.
Beef, roast	4 slices
Potatoes, mashed	½ cup
Green Beans	¼ cup
Bread, white	1 slice
Butter	
for beans	1 tsp.
for potatoes	1 tbs.
for bread	1½ tsp.

Late-Evening Snacks
Coffee	2 cups
Milk	¼ cup
Sugar	2 heaping tsps.

Other
Aspirin	2	at noon

Although the foods *you* eat and their quantities will differ, the above example indicates the preciseness necessary for you to complete your dietary analysis. Don't be sloppy; try to be as exact and accurate as possible. Remember—if you leave something out, the dietary analysis will be incorrect and will be of little help when you try to knock off those extra pounds. Be certain to include water, medications, chewing gum, cigarettes, and any other food you put into your mouth. Take note of any symptoms you may experience during the day. You'd be surprised at how many people have frequent headaches, take medication for them almost daily, and yet when asked if anything is bothering them, answer in the negative.

One particularly amusing (and personally embarrassing) story regarding this seemingly unimportant trait, is relevant:

A gentlemen sought me out not only to lose weight, but also because he just didn't feel good. He felt bloated and puffy, had been to another physician, and had undergone a complete physical examination only to be told that there was nothing wrong with him, except for being slightly overweight. Since he continued to feel poorly, he finally decided to do something about his weight.

When I first saw him, I immediately knew something was wrong. His hands and feet were puffy and he had a mild facial pallor. I requested results of his recent examinations, and advised him to do a dietary analysis until I could get back to him. Before treating him, I wanted to know exactly what his other doctor had found.

Five days later he returned to my office. I was just about to tell him that his previous doctor had performed all the indicated tests when I noticed a suspicious notation on his dietary analysis. On each of the previous three days, this man had listed, under "Other," anywhere from two to four doses of a popular alkalizer. Yet, when I first glanced at his dietary sheets, I hadn't noticed anything written under Symptoms.

I was about to discharge this apparently unhealthy gentleman because neither his examinations nor dietary analysis revealed any reason for his puffiness and bloated feeling.

But suddenly, the reason for his puffiness was there, right in front of me, neatly printed on each page of the analysis.

I asked him why he was taking so much alkalizer. He replied;

"No reason, I just like it."

After several minutes of talking, I discovered that this man had been taking an average of two daily doses of this potent medication, every day for the past eighteen months. He had started taking it to relieve headaches that he knew were caused by too much alcohol and not enough sleep. But he had continued taking it, even in the absence of any discomfort, for almost a year and a half.

I learned that during a particularly strenuous few weeks, while this man was campaigning for a local political office, he had begun drinking too much alcohol on a daily basis. To relieve the effects of his impropriety, he had started taking this medication. Fortunately, after he was elected, he refrained from drinking more alcohol than his body could reasonably handle. Unfortunately, he continued to take the medication. The aspirin content of this particular alkalizer, along with the alkaline medication it contained, was the cause of his puffiness. I recommended that he immediately stop taking it.

In two days the puffiness was gone, the pallor was reduced, and his weight was normal. Taking the medication had caused his body to retain large quantities of fluid, which caused him to be slightly overweight. In addition, the retained fluids had so swollen his body that he couldn't even remove his wedding band from his finger.

At the time he was discharged from my office, this fine gentlemen was effusive in his thanks. He felt better than he had in two years. The pressures of his political office, on which he had previously blamed his sluggish behavior, no longer presented a problem. He felt both energetic, enthusiastic and ready to handle the problems which faced him each day.

I have related this story because some individuals think that what they are taking in the form of over-the-counter drugs is insignificant or unimportant. Believe me, whatever you ingest has a bearing on your well-being, and I would caution you to be especially aware of the following:

A) Headache medication

B) Sinus medication

C) Allergy medication

D) Laxatives

E) Heartburn/indigestion remedies

As you fill out your dietary analysis, the above story will hopefully come to mind and assist you in becoming aware of the potency of the drugs you are taking. I certainly hope so.

How the Analysis Works

Once you have filled in your dietary sheets for three consecutive days, you will be ready to determine exactly where you stand regarding your food intake.

On separate sheets of paper, write down the following food categories: Meat, Fruit, Fat, Milk, Bread, Required Vegetable, Vegetable Desired, and Free Choices. I have found it best to use a separate sheet of paper for each category. This way you will have sufficient room to write in both the food and the quantity eaten.

Once you have done this, return to Chapter 5. Compare the food and quantities you have eaten for the past three days with the food categorie list contained in that chapter.

For example, if on the first day of your dietary analysis you had two eggs scrambled in butter for breakfast, you would find under the meat category that each egg is equal to one serving. You therefore ate two servings of meat at that first breakfast. Write two eggs on the sheet of paper that you labeled meat. Then, on the right side of the sheet, on the same line as the two eggs, write in the number two. This indicates that the two eggs are equal to two servings of meat.

Additionally, if you had used a teaspoon of butter to cook the eggs, you would notice that under the fat category you also had one serving at this meal. Therefore, on the sheet labeled fat, you would write down one teaspoon of butter. To the right, on the same line, write the number one to indicate that this amount of butter equals one serving of fat.

Continue on in this fashion for each food and each meal until you have accounted for everything you've eaten over the past three days. Don't forget medications and other items that are normally not considered food.

Once you have done this, add the number of servings in each category together. This will give you the total number of servings in each category that you have consumed in the past three days.

Next, divide each of these total servings by three (for the three days of the analysis), and you will find the *average* number of servings of each food that you consume daily.

Once you have done this, compare what you have eaten with the recommended number of servings stated in Chapter 5.

Are you eating too much? If you are, you already know the cause of your obesity—you are eating too much food. You will have a hard time denying the validity of this statement once you perform your own accurate dietary analysis.

Many obese individuals think they are eating minimal quantities of food. Once they can actually see what they've been eating, they can easily recognize what must be done.

How Janice T. Lost Pounds While
Reducing Her Blood Pressure

Janice was only thirty-eight years old when she first came to my office. She was overweight and had hypertension (high blood pressure). Yet even though she carried excess weight, I could easily see that she was a beautiful woman. Unfortunately, because of her obesity, Janice had "let herself go." I am sure that as a young woman, Janice had taken great pleasure in her beauty, but now, simply because she felt "unattractive," she had allowed herself the dubious luxury of not taking care of her appearance.

Janice had already tried taking medication for her blood pressure, but had discarded that approach because she disliked the thought of taking drugs for the rest of her life.

Her previous doctor had told her that she might be able to lower her blood pressure if she lost some weight. When Janice heard of the work I was doing with obesity, she felt that I might be able to help her.

After a complete examination and consultation, I concluded that Janice's hypertension was not being caused solely by her obesity. I ordered some special laboratory tests, and the results showed that my original suspicion was correct.

Janice was a victim of Hyperlipoproteinemia (specifically—Type 4 Endogenous hypertriglyceridemia). In the past, Janice had been advised to lower her cholesterol (fat) intake in an effort to control her hypertensive condition. Unfortunately, cholesterol consumption is not the cause of this condition, and therefore the problem had apparently gone unchecked for several years.

I asked Janice to perform a dietary analysis. Several days later, I discovered that she was not only eating too much food, but also that she was eating improperly. She was consuming only minimal amounts of fat-containing (cholesterol containing) foods (as she had been directed), but she was substituting increased quantities of carbohydrate (sugar and starch) foods in their place.

Since Type IV Hyperlipoproteinemia responds quite well to a *low* carbohydrate diet, I advised Janice to cut back on these specific foods, and told her to take a niacin supplement. Both these measures are recognized as effective treatment for this condition.

In less than two weeks, Janice had reduced her weight by nine pounds, and her blood pressure was within normal limits.

The simple expedient of altering only a portion of her normal dietary intake had given her the results she had been seeking. With her blood pressure reduced and the pounds coming off, Janice exhibited a new interest in life; specifically in her appearance.

She started herself on a program of increased awareness. In only a few weeks, the woman who originally had visited me no longer existed. Janice had bought new and attractive clothes and had visited her hairdresser, who transformed the almost totally gray, limp hair style she had worn on her first visit, into a chic and strikingly beautiful coiffure.

Janice was a new woman. She was proud of who she was, and by her actions and outward appearance, she showed the world her renewed pride in her appearance.

It took several months for Janice to reach her weight-loss goal, but she did it with a certain flair that I have rarely seen in overweight patients.

To be sure, Janice's case is not unusual, and it illustrates why a complete physical examination is essential before altering your food intake. I have recorded Janice's experiences in order to stress the importance of proper health care, and also to show you how easily *you* can lose weight by following the recommendations in this chapter.

How to Use the No-Diet Diet With the Super 500 Program

Once you have performed a dietary analysis, you can immediately see the kind and quantity of food you generally eat. To lose weight, you need only gradually reduce the number of servings of each food category.

In the above example, in which I was showing you how to perform a dietary analysis, I stated that on the first morning of recording your food intake, you consumed two scrambled eggs. By simply refraining from having two eggs and instead eating only one, you can immediately reduce your daily meat intake by one complete serving.

Instead of having your egg scrambled, you might enjoy a soft-cooked or poached egg. By having it this way, you immediately reduce your intake of fats by one serving, since you eliminate the butter to scramble the eggs.

As you can see, it isn't very difficult to reduce your food intake once you are aware of the amounts you are eating. As I mentioned earlier, you should reduce the quantity of foods eaten on a gradual basis. Don't try to cut back on your intake too severely; take your time and you won't even notice that you are eating less. Your scale, however, will begin reflecting your weight loss.

At the same time, it is important that you not alter the quality of the foods you eat, since doing so will most likely result in your craving these foods, with the end result being that you once again find yourself "cheating" on the diet. A reasonable approach to this method of weight loss is as follows:

1) On the first day of dieting, eliminate a single serving of fat from your intake. This may be in the form of butter normally used on your bread or vegetables, in cooking, or from another area.

2) On the second day, eliminate one meat serving.

3) Maintain this level of food intake for one week. At the end of this time, reevaluate your fat intake; if it is still excessive, reduce it by another serving.

4) The following day, if your meat intake is still too high, reduce that area by one serving.

5) Continue in this fashion, adjusting your intake downward once a week.

6) When you have reduced your intake of fats and meats to the recommended levels, you should then begin cutting down on the milk and bread categories in the same fashion.

7) Once you have reduced your intake in these four categories, you can then evaluate your consumption of fruits and vegetables.

You should not reduce your intake of these food categories until last, since they serve to maintain adequate bulk in the digestive tract. By eliminating fruits and vegetables early on, you may find that constipation and bloating occur. If your fruit and vegetable intake is only slightly more than is recommended, you need not reduce these categories at all.

As you can see from the above list, a reduction of all food categories takes several weeks. This is intentional, and has been proven to be the best and easiest way to reduce your food intake.

Don't be in a hurry: this method of weight reduction has been called the "No-Diet Diet" because you will hardly know you are dieting. As I mentioned before, this method will take a considerable period of time to reflect your ideal weight, but its good points far outweigh any disadvantages it may have regarding the length of time required.

Secondly, I know of no contraindication to losing weight in this fashion. If you are overweight and bothered by some physical ailment, the "No-Diet Diet" can, and should, be used to limit your intake of food.

Don't forget to consult with your family physician, though. He or she is the only person qualified to advise you on the status of your personal health. I have heard the complaints of numerous patients, each of whom felt that their own doctors didn't care or wouldn't take the time necessary to consult with them. I realize that although this may be true in some instances, there is no better alternative. If you are adamant in your demand for better and more personal health care, you will receive it. If you permit yourself to be ignored or otherwise disregarded, you have only yourself to blame.

How to Lose "Slow and Easy"

I have found that some patients, and especially women, require a longer period of time to adjust to new diets. If you notice a craving to once again increase your consumption of various foods, do not be concerned.

Instead of remaining in a stress-producing situation, simply increase the amounts of food until you are satisfied. At that time, if you are still eating less than before you performed your dietary analysis, you will continue to lose weight. If you then are satisfied and comfortable with the amount of food you are eating, don't worry about how long it takes you to achieve your ideal weight.

Too many obese individuals who are emotionally, psychologically, and most importantly, physically unprepared for the stresses associated with rapid weight loss attempt to lose all their excess weight *immediately*.

Most often, these individuals fail miserably and become disgusted with themselves. I realize that you want to be slender **now**. But if you are one of those individuals who, because of some physical or emotional factor, is unable to withstand the pressures of continuous dietary control, even for the short period of twenty-one days, don't force yourself to do something you will not enjoy.

Proceed in a slow and easy fashion, using the "No-Diet Diet" to reduce your weight. You will be amazed at how quickly you begin to notice changes, and you will enjoy every moment of your program because you need not consciously restrict your intake of food on a daily basis.

Once you have altered your consumption of specific foods for several days, the habit of eating less will be ingrained, and you won't have to pay attention to every bit of food you eat.

If you find that you crave certain foods and are only satisfied at an intake level above that which I have recommended, you needn't concern yourself either. Eat the amount that satisfies you for a few days, then eliminate a single serving of *any* (except fruits or vegetables) food.

Do nothing more for at least two weeks. Then, if an additional reduction is warranted, again reduce your intake by another serving. Continue to do this at fourteen-day intervals. You will find that by extending the amount of time between each reduction, you won't even notice the fact that you are eating less.

Don't worry about intervening parties or occasions that may come up. Even if you eat and drink more than usual at these times, you will continue to lose weight. Perhaps the "No-Diet Diet" can be equated with the fable about the hare and the tortoise. Slow and easy often gets the results that rushing around pell-mell misses.

The Plate Block, and How It Works

A simple method that has proven beneficial to many patients who want to reduce their intake of food is the plate block. The ingenuity of those patients who have used this little trick often leaves me breathless. The idea behind the plate block is to take up some room on your plate with an inedible object, thereby reducing the space available for food.

When I first suggested this to a patient, I was thinking primarily of some vegetable item such as parsley sprigs that most people don't normally eat.

Instead, she came back and told me that she used a *quarter* on her plate. Every time she sat down to fill her dish with the food from the table, she would place a dirty coin on her plate.

I was flabbergasted!

Why would anyone want to use such an unappetizing item as a plate block? But there was a method to her madness.

She rationalized that if she put something like parsley sprigs on her plate, she would most likely pile her food up on another area of the dish and therefore make no true reduction in the amount of food she was eating.

A quarter, on the other hand, was just as unappetizing to her as it was to me. By placing this item on her plate, she stimulated herself to be very careful about where and how much food she piled on the dish.

She was afraid the quarter would touch her food, and she knew she couldn't eat the food if this occured. For her, the quarter acted as the perfect plate block.

For you, however, parsley sprigs may be better. Don't dismiss this idea. I realize that you are probably telling yourself that you don't need anything like a plate block to help you reduce your intake of food, but remember, pride goeth before the fall.

Use each and every trick and idea to assist you in your campaign for slenderness, and slenderness will be easily obtained. I wouldn't suggest these unusual measures had they not proven beneficial to others.

Another method related to the plate block method that has been used successfully by a number of patients, may be of help.

Use a smaller plate! That's right, a smaller plate. Most of us use regular-sized dinner plates when we eat. There is no reason to have an overly large plate, with the resulting empty spaces that will appear once we try to cut back on our intake of food.

By utilizing a smaller dish to serve yourself, you will effectively "trick" your subconscious mind into seeing a "full" plate of food when you sit down to eat. I realize that this may seem foolish, but I guarantee that it works, and it works well.

One Serving Is Sufficient

Another simple method of reducing your food intake is to eat only a single serving of each type of food being offered.

You are probably telling yourself that most times you only have a single serving, but you are probably mistaken. What you consider to be a single serving is probably more like three servings. I have watched people pile mashed potatoes up on their plates so high, you would think they were going to ski down the side of them. It was only a single serving, but what a serving!

Don't be complacent; observe the quantities of food you are consuming—your dietary analysis is an accurate reflection of what you eat. If you realize you are taking oversized portions of a particular food, cut back. Eat a *single serving* and your excess pounds will just melt away.

Use the information contained in Chapter 5 concerning the size of each portion of food. Initially, measure the quantity of food you put on your dish. You'll be astonished by how much more you are eating than is recommended.

Once you recognize how much of each food equals a serving, you will have no difficulty limiting yourself to the proper amounts. On the other hand, if you never determine exactly how much is enough, you'll continue to eat too much.

How Jim K. Beat the Chocolate Doughnut

Jim worked in a fairly large office building in West Palm Beach for seven years. Each morning when he went to work, he would find himself having coffee and a chocolate doughnut for his mid-morning coffee break. Time and again, Jim promised himself that he would eliminate the chocolate doughnut from his diet. But every morning when the coffee wagon came by, Jim found himself craving (and ordering) a chocolate doughnut with his coffee. When I first heard of this problem, I was amused.

"Just don't order the chocolate doughnut," I advised.

But I didn't realize how much Jim craved that doughnut. After several weeks, Jim had pretty much accepted the fact that he was unable to refrain from having his favorite mid-morning snack.

To try to help him, I suggested that he bring a small knife with him to work. "Each morning," I suggested, "cut a small sliver out of the doughnut and discard it. Eat the remaining doughnut. Each day, increase the size of the sliver you discard."

"OK," Jim agreed.

For the next week Jim did as I had suggested; each morning the size of the sliver increased, and each morning Jim was eating less and less of the doughnut. During the second week, Jim stopped ordering a doughnut with his morning coffee.

"How did you do it?" I asked, when I saw him again.

"Oh, it wasn't all that hard," he responded. "By the end of that first week, I was eating less doughnut than I was throwing away. When I stopped to think about the stupidity of that fact, I decided not to waste any more money on doughnuts that were being discarded. I just stopped ordering them with my coffee."

I am sure you are thinking that Jim had more than just a weight problem, but I assure you: incorporating simple tricks like the missing doughnut sliver or plate block really does work.

If you honestly want to make weight loss a more enjoyable adventure, try one of these "tricks," or make up some of your own. You will be pleased with the results they achieve.

CHAPTER 11

HOW TO KEEP WEIGHT DOWN WHILE DINING OUT

One of the most difficult times to maintain a diet is while dining out away from home. Restaurant food, for instance, is notoriously fattening.

Because their major concern is pleasing the palate as easily and inexpensively as possible, restaurant chefs generally prepare meals that contain the least costly ingredients. The meals are then made more appealing by camouflage. Thickened sauces, sweeteners, and the addition of fats are three of the most common ways that restaurants camouflage their meals.

Similarly, when you are invited to a friend's home for dinner, you can be sure the meal contains more calories than you might care to consume. Friends and neighbors, in an effort to show that they care, often prepare elaborate and fattening meals. It is a rare occasion indeed, when you are offered simple fare at a friend's home.

Cocktails, appetizers, three or four main courses, and desserts are often what await you when you are invited to dine at another's home.

In addition to this, the occasion or event being cele-
brated often leads one to disregard what he or she knows is
right. Happy and joyous events lead to the inevitable conclusion that one will overindulge. Sad and stressful happenings are often ameliorated by an excess of food and drink.
Whether it's a wake or a wedding, there will undoubtedly be
greater temptation than one would care to resist.

How then, can you maintain your slenderness while still
enjoying the "luxury" of dining out? How can you, in all good
conscience, accept an invitation to dine with friends when
you know you won't be able to eat much of what has been
prepared?

If you are like most of us, you don't want to hurt a
friend's feelings or embarrass a dining companion. What,
then, can you do?

Eat and Enjoy!

How Diane C. Lost 27 Pounds and Still Enjoyed Herself

Diane, at age 24, was decidedly obese. Married and the
mother of two children, she just couldn't seem to lose her
excess weight. There was no question that Diane wanted to
be slender once again, but her husband's job demanded a
considerable amount of socializing. It wasn't that Diane
didn't enjoy dining out two or three times weekly. Her
personality was such that not only was she a welcome
addition to almost any gathering, but she also enjoyed
parties and good food.

"How can I possibly lose weight when I am faced with
rich and delicious foods at almost every turn? If we are not
dining with business associates, we are eating at restaurants
with friends. I just don't see how I am going to be able to lose
weight and still maintain the social schedule that Bob and I
have become accustomed to."

These were Diane's first words when she sat down in my
office, depressed and anxious.

"Don't be so negative," I scolded. "If you honestly want
to lose those excess pounds, I am sure that you and I can find
a way to do it without too much trouble."

We then discussed and analyzed her life style, eating habits, and even her daily activities. In less than an hour, we came upon what appeared to be the perfect solution. Our only concern was whether or not Diane could follow through.

In less than two months, we had our answer. Diane lost 27 pounds. It wasn't the easiest weight loss I've ever seen, but Diane maintains, to this very day, that she enjoyed herself the whole time. The "perfect solution" to Diane's obesity problem came in the form of the morning-after fast.

Prior to consulting me, Diane had always related her obesity to the fact that she did a considerable amount of entertaining. She gave little thought to the possibility that she could lose weight on those days when she didn't entertain or wasn't being entertained. The routine that Diane and I agreed upon went something like this:

1) When invited out, attending a social function, or eating in restaurants, Diane would eat and drink as she pleased.

2) The day after the socializing, however, Diane would maintain a strict water fast.

In all honesty, I wasn't certain that Diane would be able to follow the agreed upon routine, but she was superb. Most obese individuals who overindulge one night, feel so depressed and guilty the next day that they eat excessively, to "soothe their conscience." This excessive eating the next day was my major concern.

Fortunately, Diane had accepted our agreed upon routine in the right spirit. She admitted that before following my instructions, she had often felt self-pity the day after a particularly enjoyable evening. But once she was directed to eat as she pleased, once she had obtained the "doctor's approval," so to speak, she felt no guilt the next day. She realized that this was her unique approach to weight loss, and in that spirit understood that the day *after* the party was the day to lose weight.

A secondary benefit of this approach to slenderness came after several weeks of following my routine. Diane, being the intelligent woman she is, began to eat less at parties and restaurants. She didn't feel she was cheating herself of any enjoyment. Instead of gorging herself or ordering large quantities of food, Diane began to eat and order discriminately. She would choose only those items she truly desired, the foods she knew she really enjoyed.

"Why should I eat foods that really didn't entice me? I knew that tomorrow I would be fasting, and for me a fast is quite difficult. I decided that if I only ate the food I really enjoyed, and didn't overdo it, I could possibly eat one meal the following day."

That is exactly what she did. Without so much as a word to me, Diane began to cut back on the food and drink she consumed at a party or restaurant. The following day, she judged approximately how much (in terms of quantity) she had denied herself. She then put together a meal equal to the amount that she hadn't eaten the night before. In this way, Diane negated the need for a strict water fast, and yet didn't take in any more calories than had she overindulged the night before.

For Diane, the simple expedient of being directed to eat as she pleased, was sufficiently motivating. Perhaps you too could follow this routine when faced with attending a wedding, party, or other social engagement. Eat and enjoy, but the next day, fast.

The Fasting Procedure

Many people have told me that they could never fast. When I ask why, they tell me they just know they couldn't. When asked if they have ever tried to fast, the answer is invariably in the negative.

If you are sitting there this very moment, telling yourself that you are one of these individuals who could never fast, you are lying to yourself.

Fasting is a simple, easy procedure. When done for only thirty-two hours, fasting (as I and most of my patients have found) is easier than dieting. Don't allow your prejudices to prevent you from trying this excellent method of weight control.

If you initiate a fast properly, you will have absolutely no problem following through. As I mention elsewhere, many obese individuals skip eating breakfast. If you do, the first time you'll even know you're fasting will be at lunch time. You'll already be about half way through your fasting procedure before you're even aware that you're fasting.

In truth, a thirty-two-hour fast, for someone who doesn't normally eat breakfast, requires only about an eleven-hour denial of food.

This is how the time breaks down:

1) The fast is begun at bedtime, so you will have absolutely no difficulty the first evening.

2) By the time you awaken in the morning, you will have already fasted for eight to ten hours. That's 25 percent of the total fasting time, and you weren't even awake.

3) If you don't normally eat breakfast, you will not be faced with the necessity of denying food until the lunch hour.

4) Assuming lunch time is at noon, you will have already fasted for approximately thirteen hours (bedtime the night before is calculated at 11:00 pm).

5) Therefore, you need only fast until bedtime. This is only eleven hours away, and only a very unmotivated individual would find it impossible to fast for those eleven hours.

6) Once you go to bed again, the fast continues throughout the sleeping hours. Once again, you are not even aware that you are fasting.

7) Thus, when you awaken the following morning, you will have gone without food for approximately thirty-two hours during only sixteen of which you were awake.

8) If you can refrain from eating breakfast that second morning, you will increase your fasting time by an additional five hours.

9) I think you'll agree that it's not really all that bad, especially when you consider the fact that you can

reduce your weight by as much as four pounds in those thirty-two hours.

I suggest that if you have never tried to fast, take this opportunity to find out how truly easy it is. Don't let yourself be "hoodwinked" into believing that a fast is some onerous duty that only a fanatical health-nut can accomplish.

On the day of the fast, consume nothing but water. You will find that your appetite won't be stimulated and you won't feel any excessive desire for food.

The biggest problem for coffee drinkers is, that while fasting, they just can't seem to get going. Looking at this another way, though, you might consider how dependent your body has become on the caffeine contained in that coffee.

Another question (objection?) that often comes up, concerns itself with the fact that many dieters get a headache if they miss a meal. I agree; most dieters will suffer from headaches when first attempting to fast. This is not always the case, but for those individuals who do react this way, take an aspirin.

Don't rationalize that a little headache is going to stop you from losing those excess pounds.

How to Incorporate Restaurant Meals Into a Slender Life Style

The major point to remember when eating in restaurants is, "I am the customer, and the customer is always right."

This may sound like some outdated proverb, but if you keep it in mind, you will have no problem maintaining your weight while eating out.

In talking to a great number of patients, who often eat at restaurants, because of their work or other commitments, I found that many felt obliged to please the waiter, cook or chef. Some of these individuals eat as many as two and sometimes three meals daily at restaurants.

When I first discovered this, I couldn't believe it. Why would patrons feel obliged to please the restauranteur? It didn't make sense (and it still doesn't), but it is a fact.

I have often observed, and I am sure you have also seen, someone quickly scan a menu while the waiter hovers over the table. Finally, the customer orders. But the order is more of a request, and it sounds like the customer really doesn't want what he has just ordered.

"Ohhh, I don't know. Let me have the steak, I guess."

Does that sound familiar? It should, because almost everyone I have ever known has said something like it at one time or another.

I have watched people in restaurants actually become tense when faced with the necessity of ordering. It appears that they don't really know what they want, but because the waiter or waitress is impatiently standing at the table, they'll order something, anything, just to get out from under the pressure. But don't *you* do that!

When you order, be sure you want what you are asking for. If all you feel like having is a cup of coffee, don't order bacon and eggs with it. If you want a small salad, say so. Don't order more than you really want, just to please the waiter.

I am sure the waiter would like you to order something that is expensive. Let's face it, most people leave a percentage of the tab as a tip, and the larger the tab, the bigger the tip. But the waiter's income is not your concern. Think first of yourself, and what you feel like eating, then you won't feel obliged to order more than you really need.

A second point to remember is, *study* the menu. Imagine the taste of the food you are considering, before you order it. Take a few moments; don't rush. You will probably find that something you were just about to order no longer holds any appeal. I have done this many times myself. I'll quickly scan a menu and almost immediately be ready to order:

"Yes," I am saying to myself, "I'll have a bowl of New England clam chowder, the rib eye steak, french fries, and a half carafe of wine."

When I stop to consider my choices, I realize that a bowl of soup may be more than I really care for. A cup of chowder will do just fine. It's the flavor of the clam chowder that I enjoy, not the quantity of liquid I consume. By the same token, the rib eye steak may not be what I really want, but if the waiter is standing at the table I'll probably order it. The fries are an automatic.

Unless I take my time to consider my choices, I know that I will fall into the same trap of ordering more than is really necessary. A half carafe of wine can be reduced to a glass. If I want more, I can always order another glass; but if I order the half carafe, I know I'll drink it all. What I am trying to point out here is that I, too, find myself being intimidated by a waiter or waitress.

The way I handle this situation is as follows: when the waiter first comes to my table for the cocktail order, I invariably refuse anything to drink. I then take my time to study the menu. I consider everything that is offered; I never entertain a preconceived notion of what I am going to eat. If the waiter returns before I am finished examining the menu, I tell him I am not yet ready to order. If he stands by the table, I ask him to give me several minutes to decide. If he just stands there—I tell him to "get lost."

"I'd appreciate it if you would give me a few minutes more to make up my mind. Please don't stand there waiting for me, it makes me uncomfortable."

Perhaps it's not the same as telling him to "get lost," but it achieves its purpose. And, it give me the time I want to make a correct decision.

If, after studying the menu, I decide that I would enjoy a cocktail before dinner, I feel no compunction about telling the waiter I have changed my mind. His reaction to this deferred request for a drink often determines the size of his tip. If he appears disgruntled, you can be sure I will let him know I do not appreciate his attitude.

In any event, the point I am making is, don't be rushed or intimidated. Don't order something you don't really want, or more than you need to feel satisfied. In a word, **think.**

Another point to remember when dining in restaurants is to consider the ingredients in the food you are ordering. You are intelligent enough to know that meat covered with a cream sauce, for instance, contains more calories than the meat alone. If you can do without the sauce, order the meat plain. Don't just accept what is on the menu; alter the food order to meet your requirements.

If you will follow these recommendations and incorporate a fast into your routine when you know you have overdone it the night before, you will have no problems eating out, whether it be at restaurants or a friend's home. You will still lose weight or maintain your slenderness.

How to Analyze a Typical Menu

Always keeping in mind the above admonition to take your time, you may still find that your restaurant experiences are too fattening. If this is your problem, you may not understand the importance of properly analyzing a menu's contents.

As a brief course in menu analysis, let's see if I can give you some pointers.

1) Always refuse a cocktail before the meal. Alcohol diminishes your natural ability to refrain from overeating. Make this a standing rule. Once you have attained your desirable weight, you may occasionally want to have a pre-dinner drink. If so, go ahead and enjoy yourself, but remember: tomorrow you will have to fast if you overdo it tonight.

2) I recommend that most dieters skip soups and appetizers. However: if, after imagining the flavor of the food you're considering, you still wish to have one of these preludes to dinner, go to it. My suggestion, however, is to try to choose the soup or appetizer that contains the fewest calories. Manhattan clam chowder, for instance, has very few calories when compared with New England style chowder. A salad, with the dressing you prefer on the side, so you can put only as much on as you really need, can be a much better choice than a Caesar Salad. Let's face it, raw eggs aren't really all that appetizing. A tomato juice cocktail, with plenty of freshly squeezed lemon juice, is an excellent choice of appetizer.

3) When ordering your entree, try to choose meat, fish, or poultry that contains the fewest extra ingredients. Added fats, creams, breadcrumbs, etc. can be done without. They only serve to diminish the flavor of the

entree, or alter it sufficiently so you may not even be sure of what you're eating. Fewer calories is the name of the game.

4) Always, and I mean always, refuse potatoes. Not because they aren't an excellent source of vitamins and minerals, but because all the goodies that you (or the chef) adds to them makes them unacceptable when you are trying to lose weight. Instead of potatoes, if you feel you will still be hungry after the meal, substitute a second serving of vegetables, or a salad.

5) Desserts are a "no-no." There is just no way to incorporate restaurant-style desserts into a diet (unless of course we're considering a Chinese restaurant: fortune cookies are OK).

6) If all else fails and you are unsure of how to order a proper meal that is compatible with weight loss or weight maintenance, simply remember that unadulterated vegetables, without additional ingredients, are always your best bet and should be your first choice. Vegetables generally contain fewer calories than any other item on the menu. They are always an excellent base for any meal. If more people would choose their vegetables with as much care as they do their entrees, there would be little need for dieting.

In conclusion, then, I would caution you to pay specific attention to the foods you choose, as well as to the quantities you order when dining out. Don't be resigned to the "fact" that you can't enjoy yourself while dieting.

An enjoyable restaurant meal can be both fulfilling and filling, without being fattening.

CHAPTER 12
USING FAST FOODS FOR FAST WEIGHT LOSS

Today's life style is such that almost every individual in the nation, at one time or another, has eaten in a fast food establishment. The constant rush of everyday life, the disappearance of neighborhood gathering places, and the continuing changes that are occuring in family structure, are at least partially responsible for this fact.

At the same time, there are numerous individuals who consider the quality and taste of food served in these establishments as excellent. For whatever reason, fast food establishments have become a part of the American life style; they literally dot the landscape.

If you thought that, until now, you could not lose weight because the foods served in these fast food establishments, and your repetitive consumption of them prevented it, take heart. There is absolutely no reason to deny yourself the pleasure of eating these foods.

If you will take the few minutes necessary to determine what and how much of the foods you are permitted, you should not have any problems incorporating fast foods into your diet.

When I refer to "how much" of these foods you are permitted to eat, I am specifically talking about how many or what size portions you should consider. Every fast food establishment that I know of uses portion control (pre-measured quantities of food) when formulating their menus. Since the food serving sizes are already determined, your only responsibility lies in the ability to restrict the number of portions you consume.

Burgers Are Great and Nutritious Too

Although I don't have any statistics to prove it, I feel that the best selling item offered by fast food restaurants is the "lowly" hamburger. Of course when you finally get to eat this juicy morsel, it no longer resembles the lowly thing it started out to be. With added flavorings, crisp, fresh vegetables, spices and herbs, that minimally respected piece of chopped beef becomes a super taste treat in the minds of millions.

If you enjoy this number-one, best selling item, you should know that it can be very nutritious, and an excellent source of protein and minerals.

The hamburger should not be considered a poor substitute for a "proper" meal. When eaten judiciously and in proper combination with other foods, burgers can become the nucleus of a properly balanced diet. Don't let the die-hards who pooh-pooh the value of fast foods dissuade you from your enjoyment of these items.

Balance your intake, and you will find that not only can you lose weight at the nearby Hamburger Heaven, but you can also do yourself a service in the form of better nutrition.

I have formulated the following material in an effort to assist you in choosing what foods to eat and what foods to avoid when dining at a fast food establishment. Unfortunately, I haven't been able to gather information on every fast food establishment in the country, so you will have to use your own intelligence when faced with the decision of what to eat when dining at an unlisted restaurant.

Generally, each fast food chain serves food based on "portion control." Therefore, a ¼ pound hamburger at one restaurant is essentially equal to one served by another. Of course, you must be aware that the amount of fat a burger contains is primarily responsible for the number of calories it provides. The juicier the burger, the more fat it contains.

Since most of the national fast food chains serve their burgers almost "dry," you can be assured that they contain minimal amounts of fat, at least by the time you get to eat them. Some of the smaller fast food restaurants advertise their burgers as being juicier. Beware—these burgers probably contain enormous amounts of calories in the form of animal fat. You should be aware that one ounce or one pound of fat contains twice the number of calories contained in an ounce or pound of pure meat, fish, poultry, bread, cereal, or any other non-fat food. If you have a choice when deciding to visit a fast food hamburger restaurant, choose the restaurant that serves burgers that are dry, not juicy.

The following list indicates the approximate food category servings contained in the hamburgers sold at the two major fast food franchises. These servings are correlated to the food category lists I have included in Chapter 5. To save you the trouble of having to return to that chapter, the food categories are, once again, as follows:

- (A) Meat
- (B) Fruit
- (C) Fat
- (D) Milk
- (E) Bread
- (F) Required Vegetable
- (G) Vegetable As Desired
- (H) Free Choices

Burger King

Food Category	A	B	C	D	E	F	G	H
Hamburger, Plain	1½				2			¼
Cheeseburger	2½				2			¼
Double Hamburger	3				2			¼
Whopper, Junior	2		1		2	¼	1	¼

Whopper	3		1		2½ ¼ 1 ¼
Cheese Whopper	4		1		2½ ¼ 1 ¼
Double Meat					
Whopper	6		1		2½ ¼ 1 ¼
Double Cheese					
Whopper	7		1		2½ ¼ 1 ¼

McDonald's

Food Category	A	B	C	D	E	F	G	H
Hamburger, Plain	1½				2			¼
Cheeseburger	2½				2			¼
Double Hamburger	3				2			¼
Quarter-Pounder	3				2½			¼
Quarter-Pounder with Cheese	4				2½			1
Big Mac	3		1		2½			¼

In addition to the basic or combination hamburgers listed above, most people enjoy fries and shakes with their meals.

Each Regular size order of french fried potatoes contains approximately 2 servings in category "C" (fat), and 2 servings in category "E" (bread).

Shakes vary in their caloric as well as their food value. Remember that chocolate shakes are generally highest in calories. Each regular sized shake contains approximately 1¾ servings in category "D" (milk), ½ serving in category "B" (fruit), and 2 servings in category "C" (fat). The additional calories found in shakes are the result of added sweetening.

Since sugars are not classified in any food category, the calories they add to foods are not considered to be of any benefit with regard to proper nutrition. Although sugars and sweeteners do add calories to food, and therefore inhibit weight loss, they do not contain any essential nutrients. You should try, therefore, to limit your intake of "sweets" that don't contain other, more nutritious foods.

The following chart indicates the caloric content of many foods normally eaten at hamburger restaurants. Carefully study the various items. I am sure you will be able to choose enjoyable and satisfying meals without overdoing it on the calorie end. At the same time, you should try to incorporate in the fast food meal those food categories that are essential to your continued good health.

Since it is very difficult to accurately break down the various foods contained in every item, you will have to relate the following information to the above listed foods.

A similar item that contains approximately the same number of calories as one of the foods listed above, will have approximately the same food value. You may therefore interchange a hamburger eaten at Burger King, with one eaten at Dairy Queen, Burger Chef or McDonald's. Since they each contain almost exactly the same number of calories, you can be reasonably sure they contain almost exactly the same amounts of the various food categories.

If, however, a particular item contains considerably fewer calories than other noted items (as does, for instance, the White Castle hamburger), you must assume that it also contains diminished food value. Take these alterations and differences in caloric and food value into consideration when ordering.

Burger King

Hamburger	230
Cheeseburger	305
Double Hamburger	325
Whopper, Junior	285
Whopper	635
Cheese Whopper	705
Double Meat Whopper	915
Double Cheese Whopper	985
French Fries, Regular	220
Shake	365

Burger Chef

Hamburger	250
Big Chef	530

Super Chef	535
French Fries, Regular	240
Shake	310

Dairy Queen

Brazier	250
Brazier, Bar-B-Que	285
Cheese Brazier	310
Big Brazier	505
Big Deluxe Brazier	540
Big Cheese Brazier	600
Super Brazier	855
Hot Dog	270
Chili Dog	325
Super Dog	505
Super Chili Dog	565
French Fries, Regular	200
Onion Rings	300
Fish Sandwich	350

McDonald's

Hamburger	250
Cheeseburger	310
Hamburger, Double	350
Cheeseburger, Double	410
Quarter-Pounder	415
Quarter-Pounder, with Cheese	525
Big Mac	557
French Fries, regular	215
Shake	320
Apple Pie	270
Egg McMuffin	315
Fish Sandwich	410
Hot Cakes/Butter	275
Muffin	135
Pork Sausage	235
Scrambled Eggs	175

White Castle

Hamburger	165
Cheeseburger	195
French Fries, regular	220
Onion Rings	340
Shake	215
Fish Sandwich	200

When to Visit the Pizza Palace

A few years ago, a national consumer group undertook a survey of fast food establishments. The survey was designed to elicit what a "typical" meal was composed of at each of the restaurants studied. Once the "typical" meals were formulated, an analysis of their food value was made.

Believe it or not—the most nutrition for the money was the "typical" meal eaten at your local pizza palace. It contained more nutrition in the form of vitamins and protein than any of the other fast food meals.

If you enjoy pizza, there is no reason to prohibit yourself from eating it on occasion. However, although it is extremely nutritious, it also contains a great number of calories. Therefore you should not overdo it! I have found that the best time to eat at the so-called pizza palaces is lunch time. Most patients, because of work commitments, social engagements, etc., can't afford to sit around all afternoon, eating and drinking. They have things to do. After a bite to eat, they're off to their jobs or meetings.

Conversely, at dinner time, they are usually more relaxed, have time to waste, or are not rushed. This set of circumstances produces leisurely, and often excessive eating. I caution you to be aware of your own personal life style. If you want to enjoy pizza without putting on those pounds again, eat when you don't have enormous amounts of time to "waste."

The following chart indicates the average number of calories contained in a typical pizza meal. These statistics relate to one of the larger pizza franchises, and will have to be correlated to what is normally served at the pizza restaurant you frequent.

I would like to offer another suggestion regarding dining at *any* restaurant: eat alone. I have observed that a person who eats alone often eats less. When you are engaged in conversation with another individual, you may not pay attention to what and how much you are eating. Therefore, whenever possible, eat alone.

Pizza Hut

½ of 13" Cheese Pizza:
  Thin Crust .... 850 calories
  Thick Crust..................... 900 calories
½ of 15" Cheese Pizza:
  Thin Crust ....1,150 calories
  Thick Crust ....1,200 calories
½ of 10" Cheese Pizza: (Thin Crust).... 435 calories
  with Beef ....488 calories
  with Pepperoni ....460 calories
  with Pork.......................465 calories
  Supreme ....475 calories

In terms of food categories, the above pizza meals provide the following approximate amounts:

Item	A	B	C	D	E	F	G	H
½ of 13" Cheese Pizza:								
Thin Crust..........	3		3	½	2		1	
Thick Crust.........	3		3	½	3		1	
½ of 15" Cheese Pizza:								
Thin Crust..........	4		3½	½	3½		1¼	
Thick Crust.........	4		3½	½	4½		1¼	
½ of 10" Cheese Pizza:								
(Thin Crust)	2		3	½	1½		½	
with Beef......	4		3½	½	1½		½	
with Pepperoni	3½		3½	½	1½		½	
with Pork......	3		3¼	½	1½		½	
Supreme	3½		3½	½	1½		1	

As you can see, the calories contained in ½ of a 10″ pizza are more than you should have at any one meal, unless you make some alteration in your daily food intake.

My suggestion is that you reduce your pre-pizza food intake to offset the number of calories you'll be consuming.

If you promise yourself that you will not eat as much *after* eating the pizza, you may find that you can't live up to your promise.

Reduce what you are permitted to eat before even contemplating the pizza, and then you can enjoy your favorite meal without feeling guilty. If you take the necessary precautions, you will not have overdone it.

Remember: Eat alone, and be prepared for what you will be consuming. You'll have no trouble occasionally eating at your local pizzeria without putting on those extra pounds.

How to Enjoy Fried Chicken Without Gaining Weight

What I have said above regarding pizza goes equally well for the eating of fried chicken. There is no reason you can't enjoy the crunchy flavor of Kentucky-style fried chicken if you take a simple precaution.

The only thing you must remember is the number of calories fried chicken contains. Reduce your intake of food prior to eating the fried chicken, and you'll have no trouble maintaining or reducing your weight.

I know that you have probably been faced with the problem of restricting your food intake many times in the past. This most often happens when you eat out at restaurants. Again, one of the benefits of eating at fast food establishments, therefore, is the fact that almost every one of them uses portion control.

What you eat and how much you eat at a Burger King, McDonald's, Pizza Hut, or Colonel Sanders', is essentially the same in Florida as what you would be served in California or New York. There is really no need to try to evaluate the number of calories or the amount of food contained in the meals served in different parts of the country; you can be sure the restaurant has limited your intake for you.

The only thing to consider, and the only limits you should put on yourself, is how many portions to order.

I mentioned earlier that most obese individuals find themselves eating more than they really require to feel satisfied. I believe this is especially true when eating out. When someone orders too much food at a restaurant, the normal response is to eat it all. People generally don't like to waste food they have ordered. This is even more evident once the check arrives.

It seems to be human nature to rationalize what we order by eating all of it. I am sure you can see the foolishness of this eating habit. If you will take a few minutes before ordering to determine the minimum amount of food that will satisfy you, you won't be faced with the necessity of forcing down more food than you really want.

As I mentioned before, wait a while after finishing your food to determine whether you are still hungry. Don't order dessert right away; give your body a chance to feel satisfied. You will find that by giving yourself some time before ordering additional food, you won't really want any more to eat.

Since Colonel Sanders' Kentucky Fried is, in my estimation, the most popular fast food concern dispensing chicken, I have listed the calorie content of its two most popular dinners.

Colonel Sanders' Kentucky Fried Chicken

2-piece Dinner:
(fried chicken, mashed potatoes, coleslaw, rolls):
      Original Recipe 595
      Crispy Recipe......................... 665
3-piece Dinner:
(same as above, with 3 pieces of chicken):
      Original Recipe 985
      Crispy Recipe 1,075

The following indicates the approximate food values (categories) of these same chicken dinners:

Item	Category							
	A	B	C	D	E	F	G	H
2-piece Dinner: (fried chicken, mashed potatoes, coleslaw, rolls):								
Original Recipe...	2		4	¼	3			1
Crispy Recipe	2		4¼	¼	3½			1
3-piece Dinner: (same as above, with 3 pieces of chicken):								
Original Recipe...	3		5	¼	4¼			1
Crispy Recipe	3		5¼	¼	4¾			1

Fast Foods: Their Calorie Content

In addition to burgers, pizza, and chicken, there are a number of fast food restaurants serving almost every conceivable kind of food. The following list incorporates some of the better known franchises. Please note that I have not included any "junk" foods in this list. For those of you who enjoy this kind of food, please see Chapter 13.

Items	Calories
Rustler Steak House	
Salad	15
Bleu Cheese Dressing	150
French Dressing	120
Italian Dressing	165
Thousand Island	150
Rolls:	
Butter.......................	40
Rustler	120
Twisted......................	185
Steaks:	
Rib Eye	370
Rustler (Strip) 1,100
Chopped (4 oz.).............	330
Chopped (8 oz.).............	660

T-Bone 1,530
Baked Potato 230
Pickle........................   5

Gino's

Sirloiner............................ 515
Cheese Sirloiner 610

Long John Silver's

Fish, Chips, and Coleslaw
            2-piece Dinner 950
            3-piece Dinner................1,190

Taco Bell

Burrito.............................. 350
Bell Burger.......................... 250
Enchirito 390
Frijoles............................. 230
Taco 145
Tostado.............................. 205

Arthur Treacher's

Chips 275
Coleslaw 125
Fish (2 pieces)......................... 345

NOTE: All calorie contents listed above are approximate. They have been established by means of synthesis, not analysis. Any foods that are listed under one restaurant heading, but not under another, are of approximately the same calorie value. For instance, a shake at McDonald's compares with a shake at Gino's. I have therefore not listed shakes under the Gino's heading.

Regular soft drinks (cola, root-beer, orange soda, etc.) contain approximately 125 calories. Giant (large) soft drinks contain 190 calories.

If you enjoy the foods served at fast food restaurants, there is no need to refrain from eating them. Once again, I remind you to restrict your intake of food at the meal *preceding* your eating out, and you won't have to worry about gaining weight.

CHAPTER 13

FOR THOSE WHO MUST: THE JUNK FOOD ADDICT'S DIET

One of the most common causes of dieting *failure* is the excessive restriction of food intake. Most diet programs recommend strict adherence to a prescribed regimen, one that is usually boring and tedious. I have found, though, that a too-severe approach to weight loss often leads to failure.

I am sure that if you have ever tried to lose weight in the past, you have found this to be so. The foods you crave are usually eliminated from the diet you are trying to follow, and, in short order, you find yourself with a continuous desire for foods you are not permitted to eat. Sooner or later, the craving becomes too strong and you cheat.

Once you find yourself in this situation, you most probably give up the ghost, so to speak. You feel guilty; you're a failure (at least at dieting).

This no longer needs to be true. I have successfully treated too many patients, especially those who enjoyed what is commonly referred to as junk food, to be persuaded to tell you that just because you "love" junk food, you can't lose weight.

The approach most commonly suggested to obese individuals by other doctors and "diet specialists," is "Break your habit. Stop being a junk-food addict!"

I strongly disagree with this approach to weight loss, and for the true junkie, it is an almost impossible order to follow.

When you attempt to lose weight, there is enough stress involved without trying to break a habit or deny your cravings. If your desire for junk food can be incorporated into a weight-reduction procedure without reducing its effectiveness, there is no reason to give up the foods you love.

How Laura Beat the "Munchies"

Laura had tried to lose weight almost every day of her adult life. Since puberty, her weight had gradually and steadily increased. The more she attempted to reduce, the more she seemed to gain. At 32 years of age, Laura was, in a word, "fat." She knew it and she had almost come to accept it as an inevitable part of her life.

When she first came to see me, it was with a feeling of despair. Laura really didn't believe I could help her. Why should she? No one else seemed capable of aiding her in losing weight.

After three consecutive consultations, I formulated a plan which I felt would work for Laura. I had discovered that she was a *continuous* eater. She didn't always overdo it at any one meal, but she was always eating *something*.

I advised Laura to record her feelings about food. I further recommended that she keep track of when and where she noticed her cravings. I explained that, for the next two days, she needn't worry about her eating habits. All she had to do was make note of what and how much she ate. Most importantly, I told her to be sure to record the time of day when she began to recognize particular desires for food.

A few days later, Laura returned to the office with a complete diary of her eating habits. It was atrocious. What I had first suspected was true. Laura never stopped eating, except during sleep.

Her day went something like this: On arising, she wouldn't eat breakfast, but instead would have a glass of soda. When she arrived at her job, she would stop at a nearby diner, and get a coffee and danish to go. Before ten o'clock, she would already be muching on candy, gum, or some other little tidbit. Shortly after ten, the coffee wagon made its rounds and Laura would have another cup of coffee and a doughnut.

At lunchtime, she would "deny" herself, and order a diet special (usually some cottage cheese with fruit salad or a hamburger pattie).

By one-thirty in the afternoon, she was again eating peanuts or chewing gum. The afternoon coffee break was a duplicate of the morning's. Before leaving the office, she would stuff another piece of gum into her mouth, "for the long, twenty-minute ride home."

Dinner was usually light, but was always washed down with grape juice ("It's better than drinking soda," she rationalized). After dinner, Laura continued to eat. Before bedtime, she would consume one or two pieces of fruit, some pretzels, peanuts, or a piece of cake.

Laura was an eating machine!

Because of her previous failures to lose weight, I felt it would be necessary to allow Laura to continue in her normal eating pattern. Any restriction on the number of times she could munch on something would, I believed, cause additional stress. Failure would be the ultimate result.

I gave Laura a list of junk foods that she could eat. I explained that she could eat as much or as little of any of the foods listed, as long as the total intake for the day didn't exceed 300 calories.

In addition, I told her to begin on the Super 500 Program, but to eliminate the satisfiers. These would be replaced by the junk foods she was permitted to munch.

By the end of the first week, Laura dropped 18 pounds. By the end of her program, some three-and-a-half months later, she had reduced her weight by 63 pounds. She was, to say the least, quite impressed with her progress.

The secret to Laura's success lay in her ability to continue to eat in the manner to which she was accustomed. By permitting several snacks during the day, I had effectively eliminated the cause of Laura's previous failures—the additional stress that resulted from her not being able to keep her mouth going continuously.

As I stated above, if you crave junk foods, you need not feel you'll never lose weight. Follow the suggestions in this chapter, and you will find the pounds melting faster than you might think.

Preparation Is the Key to Success

The boy scout motto, "Be prepared," is a good one for dieters. If you would like to lose those excess pounds, but know you will crave "goodies," you must be prepared.

The simplest suggestion is to formulate a list of the snacks and goodies you will probably want to eat during a full day. Then, prepare these snacks into individual serving sizes using the list I have included below. Just be sure that the total intake for the day doesn't exceed 300 calories.

Once you have the proper portions set aside, promise yourself that you will eat nothing else other than the meals permitted in the Super 500 Program that day. That's really all there is to it.

If you have decided to chew several pieces of gum during the day, don't take the entire pack with you. Separate the correct number of pieces, and put the rest away, out of sight. If you will be eating jelly beans, measure them out, wrap them in plastic, and put the remainder away. Do this for each and every snack and junk food.

Don't think that once you start muching you'll be able to control the amount of food you consume. If you have the correct amount at your disposal, you won't be tempted to overdo it. You'll eat just the right amount, not more or less.

If you go to work, take the "goodies" along in your purse or pocket. Put them out of sight (and partially out of mind). When you feel like having something, don't hesitate. Eat one or more of the snacks you've prepared. You needn't feel guilty, or that you are cheating; you are eating precisely what is indicated in your diet program. Enjoy yourself, but remember, nothing is to be eaten in excess of the pre-measured snacks.

You'll lose weight and have a great time doing it. You'll be amused by the stares of those around you when you tell them you are dieting, while eating your favorite junk foods.

Suggestions Which Have Helped Others

In addition to the caution about preparing your snacks in advance, there are two suggestions I would like to make.

First, don't eat impulsively. It's fine to eat your snacks when you notice a craving, but don't disregard the need to be aware of what you eat. Some patients who have used the "Junk Food Addict's Diet," reported that the amount of goodies they were permitted to eat was inconsequential. Once I stressed the importance of being conscious of the snacks they were eating, all complaints ceased.

These dieters had been eating impulsively. They were not aware of what or how much they were consuming. It is easy to fall into the trap of thinking you still have a craving for additional snacks, if you don't pay attention to everything you're eating. Once you recognize that you just finished a snack, the "munchies," or cravings for additional foods, generally subside.

You will probably experience the same feelings that my patients reported. Once you pay attention to what you are permitted to eat, however, you will agree that it is more than enough to quell your cravings for junk food.

Second, I must stress that, initially, you should choose the junk foods with the fewest number of calories. You are still permitted to consume 300 calories a day in junk food, but by choosing lower calorie foods, you will be able to have several additional snacks during the day, if you so desire.

Instead of trying to limit your snacks to one or two, prepare a list of six or seven snacks. By putting chewing gum and popcorn on your list, you will be able to indulge yourself more frequently during the day.

Once you have become comfortable with the way the "Junk Food Addict's Diet" is proceeding, you can replace some of the lower-calorie foods with those you crave more. As long as you keep the snack limit to within 300 calories, you'll have no problem.

If you give yourself an opportunity to become accustomed to the snacking procedure by choosing lower-calorie foods, you won't produce the additional stress that results from having to limit yourself to only a few snacks a day. You'll find that once you follow these recommendations for several days, you won't have the frequency of cravings you did initially. At that time, you may choose the junk foods you desire.

How to Set Up Your Snack Times

Before beginning on the "Junk Food Addict's Diet," you should make note of how often you crave food. What I did for Laura, you should do for yourself.

Determine the amount of food you eat and the time of day you normally eat it. Note specifically how many snacks you really consume. Then, when you are ready to begin dieting, prepare at least enough snacks to meet the number of times you generally crave food.

I ordinarily suggest that you formulate a list of snacks that meet your usual needs. Then divide one or more of the food portions into two or more packages. In this way, you will be prepared for the event that you may want food more often when you begin dieting.

In the event that you don't crave additional snacks, you can either eat or discard the excess food you've packaged. If you discard it, you will, of course, find that you lose weight faster than anticipated.

How Sheila K. Lost 106 Pounds While Eating Potato Chips and French Fries

Sheila had spent her childhood in a small Georgia town. Her normal diet consisted of large amounts of pork, pork fat, and fried foods. When she moved to Florida at the age of 24, Sheila was already overweight.

Fortunately, many of the foods that had been served in her home were no longer readily accessible. Sheila subconsciously substituted french fried potatoes, and potato chips for the foods she missed.

Over the years, Sheila's weight increased. By the time I saw her, she was 110 pounds overweight. The strain on her heart, along with the discomfort she experienced during the Florida summers, were the motivating factors responsible for Sheila's seeking help in losing weight.

After the preliminary examination and consultation, I realized that just as Laura had craved typical "junk food," Sheila craved chips and fries. I put together a program of dieting that I felt would meet Sheila's needs. I permitted her to eat one daily serving each of french fries and potato chips. But, if she wanted to lose those extra 100 plus pounds, Sheila would have to restrict her other foods.

I made a list of foods that she would have to give up. Once she looked it over, she stated several objections. She felt that the list was too extensive, and that she would inevitably falter and cheat.

I revised the list, and submitted it once again. Now Sheila agreed! She honestly felt that she would be able to give up all the foods on the list, if she were permitted to eat the fries and chips along with other less fattening foods she craved.

Here is the list of foods that were forbidden for Sheila, and to which she and I had agreed: Any and all foods that were prepared with added fats of any kind.

Simple, wasn't it? All she had to do was eliminate all added fats from her diet. The only fats she was permitted to eat were those contained in the fries and chips.

Sheila relished her customized diet. She couldn't believe that she could eat anything she wanted (in accordance with the recommended food category lists), plus fries and chips, and still lose weight. But lo and behold, five months later, Sheila had reduced her weight to within 4 pounds of her goal. She had shed 106 pounds and was discharged from the office.

Note: When I first began to write this paragraph, Sheila had been following my diet for six weeks. At that time, she had reduced her weight by 42 pounds, and the heading of this paragraph reflected that fact. It had been entitled *How Sheila K. Lost 42 Pounds While Eating Potato Chips and Fries.*

Now, as I return to this chapter to edit and correct it, more than seven months have passed. Sheila is no longer a patient, having been discharged some four months ago after dropping an additional 64 pounds. She no longer requires any guidance I could give her.

How to Use Those Cravings to Lose Weight

I mentioned above that not giving in to your cravings results in additional stress. I honestly believe that by using your cravings constructively, you can assist yourself in losing weight.

Both Laura and Sheila had cravings for "taboo" foods. Any other diet would have prevented them from eating the foods they enjoyed, and I am sure they would have failed to achieve their goals.

If you find that you have a desire for specific foods, don't try to restrict your intake of these items. You will only be fighting a losing battle.

Instead, use your intelligence to design a customized diet that includes both the recommended food categories *and* your special junk food.

You'd be surprised at how many overweight people believe they can't lose weight because they *just* can't give up some special food they enjoy. You *can* lose weight and you *will* lose weight, if you use your cravings in a positive manner.

Don't listen to people who tell you that you *must* give up everything you enjoy if you want to be thin. "It just *ain't so.*"

How to Include Junk Foods
Without Sacrificing Weight Loss

If you will return to Chapter 5, you will find all the information necessary to formulate your daily food intake. Make yourself a list of several meals that meet the requirements of the food category lists. Be specific; don't generalize. Write out exactly what, and how much, of the various foods you'll be eating.

Next, consider the method of preparing the foods you'll be eating. Once you have done this, you will have the foundation of your own, customized, Super 500 Program.

When you have done this, return to this chapter and make a list of several junk-food snacks you enjoy. Incorporate a maximum number of low-calorie snacks into your daily food pattern. Be sure not to exceed 300 calories, though. Then, once you begin on your customized 500 program, you will know exactly what, and how much, you may eat.

That's all there is to it. It's a simple method of reducing your food intake and therefore your weight, while at the same time permitting you to eat the foods you crave.

In the following list I have tried to include most of the foods that are considered "junk"; however, I may have missed some. If you cannot find the foods you crave in this list, you might look in Chapter 12, where I have included the calorie content of fast-foods.

If you are still unable to find what you are looking for, I suggest you purchase a copy of *Composition Of Foods*, Agriculture Handbook No. 8, Agricultural Research Service, United States Department of Agriculture. You can obtain this from the Superintendent of Documents, U.S. Government Printing Office, Washington, D.C. 20402.

JUNK FOODS

Calorie Content
1. Cakes (1 piece 2″ x 2″ x 1″)

Angel Food	160
Boston Cream Pie	310
Caramel Cake	400
Chocolate Devil's Food	320
Coffee Cake	350
Fruit Cake	60
Gingerbread	370
Honey Spice Cake	365

Marble Cake	290
Pound Cake	140
Sponge Cake	200
White Cake	385
Yellow Cake	390

Note: As you can see from the above list, cakes are generally very high in calories. I would, therefore, recommend that you try to formulate your snack list without them, at least initially. If you feel that you will probably crave some cake during the day, I suggest that you either include the lowest calorie ones, or utilize only half a piece of the higher calorie ones.

2. <u>Candy</u> (1 oz.)

Butterscotch	115
Caramels	120
Chocolate, Fudge	120
Chocolate, Fudge, with Nuts	130
Chocolate Mints (1)	45
Chocolate "Tootsie" Roll	110
Gum Drops	100
Jelly Beans	105
Marshmallows	90
Milk Chocolate	145
Milk Chocolate with Nuts	155
Peanut Brittle	120
Peanut Butter Candy	130

3. <u>Cookies & Crackers</u>

Brownies (1)	95
Butter (1 oz.)	130
Chocolate Chip (1)	50
Fig Bars (1 Oz.)	100
Gingersnaps (1 oz.)	120
Ladyfingers (1)	40
Macaroons(1)	90
Marshmallow (1 oz.)	75

Molasses (1)	135
Oatmeal (1)	60
Peanut (1)	60
Sandwich-type (1 oz.)	135
Sugar Wafer (1)	40
Raisin (1)	65
Shortbread (1)	35
Vanilla Wafer (1)	20
Crackers, Graham (1)	55
Crackers, Graham, Chocolate-Coated (1)	60

4. Desserts

Chocolate Pudding (½ cup)	195
Gelatin (1 oz.)	95
Ice Cream (½ cup)	130
Ice Milk (½ cup)	100
Orange Sherbet (½ cup)	130
Tapioca Pudding (½ cup)	110

5. Drinks (1 ounce)

Cola Soda	10
Chocolate Drink	25
Cream	15
Fruit Flavored	15
Ginger Ale	10
Grape Drink	15
Grape Juice	20
Root Beer	15
Lemonade	15
Limeade	10

6. Nuts

Almonds (2)	10
Almonds, chopped (1 tbs.)	50
Brazil Nut (1)	25
Cashews (1 oz.)	160
Chestnuts (1 cup)	190
Hickory Nuts (1 oz.)	225
Macadamia (1 oz.)	230
Peanuts, Dry Roasted (1 oz.)	105
Peanuts, Regular (1 oz.)	95

Pecans (½ cup)	370
Pecans, chopped (1 tbs.)	50
Pistachios (1 oz.)	170
Walnuts (1 oz.)	180
Walnuts, chopped (¼ cup)	195

7. Other

Chewing Gum (1 stick)	5
Popcorn (1 cup)	25
Popcorn, buttered (1 cup)	40
Potato Chips (1 oz.)	160
Pretzels (1 oz.)	110

8. Pies (⅛ of a 12″ pie)

Apple	300
Banana Custard	250
Blueberry	285
Cherry	310
Chocolate Chiffon	265
Coconut Custard	270
Custard	250
Lemon Chiffon	255
Lemon Meringue	270
Mince	320
Peach	300
Pecan	430
Pineapple	210
Pineapple Chiffon	255
Pumpkin	240
Sweet Potato	245

CHAPTER 14

MELT POUNDS AWAY
WHILE PAMPERING YOURSELF

After treating hundreds of obese patients, I have come to the conclusion that strenuous exercise is not one of their favorite pastimes. Certainly it is a rare individual who *does* enjoy calisthenics or weightlifting; but she or he is the exception that proves the rule.

I realize that there are many overweights who like to take part in physical activities, but I don't consider these activities to be in the same category as *exercise*. To me, exercise is a repetitive, monotonous, and usually nonproductive set of movements. The activities that overweight individuals seem to take part in are those which, although they may be nonproductive, are enjoyable. Even though these activities often burn up more calories than regimented exercise, the participant generally sees them as being *fun*.

For instance, most overweight people shun the jogging trails; yet they are often the first ones on the dance floor at a party. With today's dances, which are often more strenuous than jogging, you can see that it is not the physical activity that is being shunned. The fact that exercises generally aren't much fun is the primary reason why obese individuals don't take part in them.

Exercise normally requires a prescribed set of movements that are unnatural, or at least uncomfortable, to perform. In addition, most exercises don't really strike the individual as being *enjoyable*.

At the same time, dancing, although it also incorporates movements that can be highly unnatural as well as uncomfortable, has a large, enthusiastic following. The only reason that I can find for this apparent enigma is that *dancing is fun*.

One of the most important factors in reducing and maintaining a slender figure is to "burn more calories than you consume." If you take a few minutes to plan your daily routine and incorporate some of the physical activities you really enjoy into your life style, you will be doing much to insure your own slenderness for life.

Don't hesitate to schedule dancing, golf, tennis, swimming, or any other activity you truly enjoy. Promise yourself that you will take part in these activities, no matter what. Don't let someone else talk you out of it.

If you enjoy dancing, make plans to do it several times weekly. Don't skimp on the activities you enjoy.

If you follow this recommendation, you'll never have to worry about doing *exercises*.

Since each individual sees different physical activities as enjoyable, I would be hard put to formulate a program of activities that would suit everyone. In addition, there are many people who don't enjoy *any* physical exertion.

For these reasons, I have incorporated into the Super 500 Program, a *nonactivity* that increases the rate at which you will burn off those pounds.

Since you will not have to take part in any "exercise," you will be able to incorporate this nonactivity into your daily routine without too much trouble. If utilized on a daily basis, this nonactivity will increase your weight loss by as much as 25 percent.

This means that whatever amount of weight you would normally lose on the Super 500 Program in four days, you will now lose in three.

Considering the fact that you don't have to "do" anything, this method, which can increase your weight loss so dramatically, is well worth your consideration.

The Easy Way to Burn Up Fat

Exercise programs produce weight loss in two ways. First, the actual exercise (movement) incorporated in the program burns up calories. Every time a muscle contracts, calories are used up. In this way, the body is forced to supply more nutrients to the muscles so they can continue their activity. Thus, muscular movement burns up calories that would otherwise be deposited in your fat reserves.

Second, the actual body movement that takes place while performing exercises produces friction, with a resultant build-up of heat within the body. This excess heat causes the metabolic rate at which the body is functioning to speed up. And, with a speed-up in the metabolic rate, there is a concomitant speed-up in the rate at which calories are burned.

Therefore, exercise programs produce weight loss by burning up additional calories over and above those normally utilized. This is the only way you can expect to increase the speed with which you lose weight.

Since exercise, per se, is rarely looked upon with affection by those who are overweight, I have designed a unique method of increasing the body's capacity to burn calories.

As I mentioned earlier, exercise forces the body to increase it's calorie utilization in two ways. Since you will not be taking part in any exercise, we cannot get your body to burn up those extra calories due to the need, of the muscle groups which are being activated, for additional nutrients.

On the other hand, there is a way to increase the body's metabolic rate without physical activity. In the previous example, I explained how exercise does this through friction. I mentioned that it was the actual *movement* that produced the increased heat, and thus resulted in an increased metabolic rate. Another method of accomplishing this is to force the body temperature to rise by some other means.

The simplest approach to accomplishing this is what I call the **Metabolic Bath**: a soothing, relaxing soak, which allows you to not only increase your metabolic rate, but to also reduce your appetite.

How Others Have Used the Metabolic Bath To Speed Up Their Weight Loss

Before giving you the specifics of how to utilize the metabolic bath, I feel it might be beneficial for you to be exposed to others' experiences with it. Since each individual's life style differs, the way the metabolic bath is incorporated also differs.

Most often, the time to enjoy this weight loss accelerator is prior to dinner. Men and women who work outside the home find a luxurious one-hour bath, just before the evening meal, to be a welcome change.

After returning home in the evening, most people are emotionally tense as well as physically depleted. To get these individuals to exercise for an hour would be nearly impossible. Yet they gladly relax in the soothing warmth of the metabolic bath.

If you work away from home, you will probably find that taking advantage of this time before dinner to soothe irritated nerves, is well worth the slight inconvenience it may produce. The fact that your normal activities may be delayed or put "out of sync" is a small price to pay for the additional pounds you will lose.

You will replenish your vitality, burn up extra calories, and, at the same time, reduce your appetite. I am sure you will find that this "soaking-time" is an exceptionally enjoyable event.

Some persons find that they can accrue the same benefits normally associated with the metabolic bath by sunbathing. Here in Florida, where the weather permits year-round outdoor activities, sunbathing is an extremely popular "nonactivity."

Fortunately, this method of increasing the body's temperature works almost as well as the metabolic bath. If you find that you have both the time and the inclination to soak up the sun's rays, please don't hesitate to use sunbathing as an excellent alternative.

Another method used by some of my patients is a steam "bath." Since these patients already had memberships at local gyms, they felt they could get at least some of their money's worth by using the steam bath facilities which were already available.

If you are presently a member of a local "health spa," you may find that you can do the same thing. In addition, if you feel energetic enough to take part in some exercise prior to the steam bath, go right ahead. Although exercise isn't essential to your weight loss, it will increase the rate at which your body burns up those extra calories.

How Allan K. Lost 62 Pounds While Relaxing

Allan was 42 years old when he first decided to do something about his weight problem. For years, he had promised himself that he would lose some weight. Unfortunately, the pounds continued to creep up on him in a gradual manner, until he could no longer ignore his obesity.

Allan's concern about professional commitments (he was a lawyer), and the years he spent actively building his practice, had left him little time to pay attention to his own health or physical appearance.

Now, at middle age, with his practice doing well, he realized he hadn't played football or basketball since college. The years he had committed to increasing his professional and financial security had somehow cheated him of the pleasures he had known as a young man, when he was involved in all kinds of sports.

Before he came to see me, Allan had attempted to lose his excess weight by following a calorie-restrictive diet and taking part in many of the sports he had enjoyed as a younger man. He reported that his physical activities no longer proved enjoyable. In fact, they were downright painful. The years Allan had spent away from sports had resulted in an enormous decline in his abilities.

Allan had become depressed. His ego, with respect to his sports skills, had been bruised. His weight had decreased slightly, but not sufficiently to make him happy with his diet. He had given up on both sports and dieting, and had returned to his sedentary ways more than 65 pounds overweight.

When I first consulted with him, I told Allan that there was no physical reason he couldn't regain his skill at sports. I recommended, however, that he put all thoughts of physical activity out of his mind for the time being. I explained the Super 500 Program to him, and also pointed out the minimum and maximum weight losses he could expect. Allan perked up!

"Isn't there something I can do to increase the speed with which I lose this excess weight?" he asked.

"Yes," I explained. "If you want to lose weight even faster than indicated by the charts, you might consider using the metabolic baths."

Allan and I discussed this approach to increased weight loss, and by the time he left my office, he had given me his verbal commitment that he would definitely try the metabolic baths.

In just six weeks, Allan had reduced his weight by 62 pounds. At 5'9", Allan now weighed 163 pounds; the lowest he had weighed since college.

Normally it would have taken at least eight weeks to achieve this goal, and considering Allan's occupation, much longer than that, yet he had done it all in exactly forty days. I was impressed!

Allan looked years younger, there was a bounce in his step, and he appeared much happier than on his first visit to my office.

At the time of his discharge, I asked Allan what he thought of the metabolic baths. I was interested in learning how he felt about this unique approach to increased weight loss. Allan explained that he was more than satisfied with the results he'd achieved, and was even happier with the

minimal amount of time it had taken. He let me in on a little
secret.

Allan revealed that while taking the metabolic baths he
didn't just relax. He told me that for the first fifteen or
twenty minutes he would close his eyes, reflect on the
happenings of the day, and allow the tension to be dissipated
from his body. After twenty minutes of this relaxed "ca-
dence" however, he couldn't take it any longer.

He started to read, listen to music (he brought a port-
able radio into the bathroom with him); he even tried to do
some work while soaking in the bath tub. No good! He was
just too restless to relax and enjoy himself.

Finally, he hit upon a solution. Allan recalled that as a
younger man, when he did get involved in sports, he always
spent fifteen or more minutes warming up before a game,
and the same amount of time cooling down afterwards.

Allan decided that, instead of doing warm-up exercises,
he would treat himself to "post-game" therapy. He started to
massage his muscles. He began with his feet, kneading the
toes, flexing the ankles. Then he would gently massage his
calves, working the tense muscles and relieving any painful
areas he found. He would continue doing this until he had
covered his entire body, revitalizing himself in the process.

After several days of this "therapy," Allan had felt limber
and ready to try his hand at sports again. Because there was
a men's softball team forming, Allan chose to try out for it.

Lo and behold, Allan made the team!

Twice a week he played softball with his new acquaintances, and twice a week his ego got a boost. The preparations
and precautions Allan had taken by limbering his muscles
up while enjoying the metabolic baths worked wonders.

Even on the day after the first softball game, Allan didn't
feel sore. The relaxed atmosphere of the bathtub, along with
the increased flexibility he had regained from his massaging
technique, helped him take part in strenuous physical activities without any untoward effects.

Not only did Allan feel better about himself, but because
he had stretched and mobilized the muscles and tendons of
his body, he performed better on the playing field. He was no
longer "hamstrung."

Allan further reported that both the metabolic baths and the involvement with sports had helped him reduce his weight faster than anticipated. In addition, he felt that both the nonactivity of the bath, and the *activity* of the softball playing, had helped him in his personal life. Softball apparently had helped reduce the stress associated with his legal practice, and the bath relieved the soreness and tension that resulted from his sometimes overdoing it on the ball field.

For Allan, the metabolic baths proved to be a superb weight loss accelerator.

Some Tips on Initiating the "Clean Machine"

As I mentioned above, most dieters prefer to take their metabolic baths just before dinner. You will have to decide whether or not this is best for you.

The main thing to remember is that you should use the metabolic bath right before a meal. If you can sunbathe, do so before lunch, not afterwards. The reason for this is that increased body heat not only increases the metabolic rate, but also reduces the appetite.

So, if you will do as I recommend, you will not only increase the speed of your weight loss, but also reduce your desire for (and intake of) food. This fact alone will accelerate your weight reduction.

To understand the proper way to enjoy the metabolic bath, you should understand the scientific reason why it functions.

Body Temperature: Its Relationship to Weight Loss

Heat is continually being produced in the body. This is the result of metabolic reactions. At the same time, heat is also being lost to the surrounding air.

When we consider the heat of the body, we must understand that we are talking about both the internal (core) temperature and the surface (skin) temperature. The internal temperature rarely varies more than one or two degrees. At the same time, the surface temperature rises and falls with the temperature of the surroundings.

Many individuals think that the measurement of body temperature, by the use of an oral or anal thermometer, is accurate and reflects the internal temperature of the body. This is not so. First, the normal temperature of the body is not 98.6°F as is commonly believed. The normal temperature of the body is a *range* of between 97°F and 99°F. Second, the temperature that is recorded by a thermometer doesn't necessarily reflect the *actual* core temperature. You must remember that the surface temperature varies according to the surrounding temperature, and that it is also a reflection of the amount of heat that must be dissipated by the internal organs.

As I mentioned above, exercise increases the internal body temperature, and it is this increase that causes a speed-up in the metabolic rate. If you remember that the core temperature of the body doesn't fluctuate by more than a degree or two, you will understand better how the body eliminates the heat generated by exercise. The body dilates the superficial blood vessels near the surface of the skin. The blood passing through these vessels is thereby cooled by the surrounding air or other material that it contacts.

Since we are not interested in exercising to increase the amount of heat that must be dissipated by the body, we must hinder the body in its attempt to release excess heat to the surroundings.

This can be accomplished by increasing the temperature of the environment surrounding the body. The metabolic bath works to achieve this.

By immersing the body in water that is adequately heated, the body's surface temperature is increased. Since it is very difficult for the body to dissipate the heat that is normally being generated by the workings of the internal organs (because it is surrounded by the heated water), the internal body temperature will rise slightly.

This rise in internal body temperature produces a reflex within the hypothalamus (the heat-control center in the brain). The body then attempts, once again, to rid itself of the excess heat.

Sweat glands are stimulated, and an increased flow of blood is diverted to the body's surface. Because the body is being hindered in its ability to dissipate the additional heat, the basal metabolic rate begins to rise. The chemical reactions that take place inside the body speed up, additional calories are burned, and additional heat is produced.

In this way, by artificially increasing the surrounding temperature of the body, we can force it to expend more energy than normal. Thus, without performing any exercise, but by simply soaking and relaxing in a tub of heated water, we can produce a more rapid weight loss.

When you first attempt to use the metabolic bath, you should be careful how hot you make it. I would recommend using a thermometer the first few times. This will give you an idea of how much you are altering your body's surrounding temperature. Start with a bath that is approximately 94°F. This bath temperature will increase your body temperature by approximately one degree, and produce a 25 percent increase in the rate of metabolism.

Please note: You should not stay too long in the bath when first using this procedure. Twenty minutes is sufficient. After you have become accustomed to your body's response to this artificially-induced heat build-up, you will be able to increase both the amount of time you spend in the bath (never exceed one hour) and the temperature of the water. The longer you remain in the bath, and the higher the temperature, the better the results will be.

I would like to caution you to not permit your body to return to its normal temperature too quickly. This sometimes causes a weak feeling, but more important, it almost always increases your appetite.

When you leave the bath, wrap yourself well in a large towel or robe. Relax in an area that is not too cool, and prolong the amount of time it takes for you to cool off. You will be surprised how this prevents your desire for food from being stimulated.

If you will be using sunbathing as an alternative to the metabolic bath, I suggest that you do your bathing in an area that doesn't allow the wind to cool you. Your body will attempt to dissipate the heat being applied to it by the sun by perspiring. If you can somehow inhibit the evaporation of the perspiration from the skin, you will have gained the same result as with the metabolic bath.

Remember, the increased body temperature will increase the rate of metabolism and decrease the appetite.

Caution: As I mentioned above, you should initially spend only a short time (twenty minutes) in this non-activity. Once you have become accustomed to the way your body responds to the inhibition of heat dissipation, you can extend your time.

Once you have adequately increased your body's temperature, you should seek a shaded area, wrap yourself well in a terry cloth robe, and allow your body to gradually return to its normal temperature.

Don't forget that if you permit a rapid return to normal temperature, you will be stimulating your appetite. That's something we don't want to do.

CHAPTER 15

HOW TO BEAT DIETER'S DEPRESSION

One of the most common problems among dieters has come to be known as dieters' depression. This condition most often results from lowered blood sugar. When one is dieting, there is a tendency to feel depressed or weakened. This, as I have said, is due to a lowered amount of sugar circulating in the blood.

On the Super 500 Program, there is little danger of ever experiencing this phenomenon. The satisfiers are designed to offset any depression since they contain adequate sugars and will increase and maintain adequate blood-sugar levels between meals. This action of the satisfiers has been explained in previous chapters.

Sometimes, because of unforeseen circumstances, a dieter is unable to take a satisfier. When this occurs, there is a possibility that depression and weakness will result.

To prevent this from occurring, I have incorporated a simple tablet into the Super 500 Program. This tablet will not only increase the amount of circulating blood sugar and increase one's energy levels, it will also reduce any cravings for sweets you may have previously experienced on other diets.

I have been both surprised and excited by the fact that a simple tablet, available at any health food store, can offset the desire for sweets, maintain sufficiently high blood-sugar levels, and generally assist every dieter in meeting the demands of weight reduction.

The Super 500 Energizer and How It Works

I have called this tablet the Super 500 Energizer not because I discovered or invented it, but because, when it is used in conjunction with the *Super 500 Rapid Weight Loss Program*, it acts to increase the dieter's energy levels, reduce fatigue, and generally eliminate the depression that may be associated with a reduction of circulating blood sugar.

Since it is not always possible to eat the satisfiers which I have listed, it is essential that you have some method of preventing low blood sugar from disrupting your diet.

Although the satisfiers were designed to do this, you may, from time to time, find it impossible to use these natural energizers.

Therefore, before beginning on your twenty-one-day program, I suggest that you obtain a sufficient quantity of these Energizers.

Go to your nearby health food store and get a minimum of 100 tablets of **fructose**. Each tablet should contain exactly two grams of fructose.

Fructose is a naturally-occuring sugar. It is found in every fruit and vegetable, and it is for this reason that it is called fructose, which means fruit sugar.

Fructose is the sweetest of all the commonly available sugars. It is sweeter than sucrose (table sugar) because sucrose is nothing more than a combination of fructose and the less-sweet glucose (another type of sugar).

Honey, for example, is primarily composed of fructose. That is the reason for its extra sweetness.

In addition to being sweeter than all the other sugars, fructose is also more slowly absorbed into the bloodstream. If we were to consider the absorption rate of glucose to be 100, fructose would have an absorption rate of only 43. This means that when you ingest fructose, it will be more slowly absorbed, and, therefore, will not produce an excessive "alimentary hyperglycemia" (increased blood sugar resulting from foods that have been eaten).

In this way, fructose, taken as directed, will gradually increase the blood-sugar levels. It will increase energy and offset any depression you may experience because of decreased blood-sugar levels.

At the same time, since it is slowly absorbed, it will increase your energy levels over a longer period of time. Also, since there is no rapid rise in the circulating blood sugar, there won't be any rebound effect. This is the letdown many individuals experience, an hour or two after they have eaten "sweets."

In all, fructose (the Super 500 Energizer) has numerous advantages over other sweets you may normally eat. It will adequately increase blood-sugar levels, decrease cravings for sweets, and offset dieters' depression. During your twenty-one-day program, if you should find that you are unable to eat the satisfiers, or if you experience a period of weakness or depression, just pop one or two of these energizing tablets into your mouth and suck or chew on them.

You will find that in a short period of time, the weakness or depression will disappear.

Another important advantage of fructose is found in its greater sweetness. Because it is so sweet, fructose can be taken in smaller quantities than other sugars. You will therefore get the same satisfying effect from fructose as you would normally get from almost twice as much of the other sugars. This means that you can use fructose more freely, without being overly concerned with its calorie content.

Four grams of fructose (two tablets) contain only about sixteen calories, yet they are as sweet as seven grams of table sugar. You will, therefore, be able to satisfy your "sweet tooth" with only about half as much sweets. This, you can see, is a decided benefit.

Satiety: the Extra Bonus

Many dieters, simply because they must pay attention to the foods they are eating while on a diet, seem to crave additional amounts of food.

Normally they would be more than satisfied with the quantity of food they are permitted to eat, but, because they are "forced" to limit their intake, they seem to respond with greater cravings for food.

By taking the Super 500 Energizer when you feel "hungry," the cravings for extra food will be offset. The few calories contained in the tablets are insignificant when compared to the calories in a doughnut or other "snack."

If you feel a desire for additional food, or if you are concerned about eating too much at the next meal, suck or chew on a few Super 500 Energizers (fructose tablets). You will be quite pleased with the results.

If taken as directed, you will not only eliminate your craving for sweets, but you will also satisfy your desire for food generally. By the time the next meal rolls around, you may find yourself eating less than usual, and without any feeling of being denied.

I recommend that all dieting patients carry with them a full day's supply of these tablets. Ten or twelve are usually sufficient. Every time you feel the need to eat a piece of candy or otherwise cheat on your diet, just pop a few of these sweet, clean-tasting tablets into your mouth.

A word of caution, though: do not postpone taking the fructose tablets. Because they are more slowly absorbed into the bloodstream, you may find yourself eating additional sweets long before the fructose has had a chance to do its job.

When you first become aware of even the slightest urge to indulge in some "forbidden" goodies, suck on a few of these tablets. In this way you will prevent yourself from experiencing a full-fledged "sugar fit." Remember, fructose takes longer to bring the blood-sugar levels up, so you must take it well in advance of having true cravings.

Once again: do not put off taking the fructose. You won't be helping yourself. I realize that you probably try to restrict yourself when dieting and often postpone eating extra food for as long as possible. But when it comes to the Super 500 Energizer, this is uncalled for and will not benefit you in any way.

Using the Energizer to Reap Maximum Benefits

Some of my patients have become so enthused about the use of the Super 500 Energizer, that they have formulated numerous ways to use these tablets to increase their weight loss.

One patient who often found it impossible to eat regular meals used the Energizer tablets as a substitute. She would take as many as ten or twelve tablets to offset the effects of a missed meal. If you think about it, ten tablets contain only eighty calories. This is much fewer than would be contained in even the smallest snack. Yet, because the fructose is absorbed slowly, this patient reported from time to time when she was forced to miss a meal, the Energizers more than controlled her appetite.

In effect, she was "skipping" a meal, and didn't even notice. The fructose maintained her energy levels and satisfied her need for food. All this on only eighty to ninety-six calories.

Another patient that comes to mind used the Energizer tablets as a replacement for all the satisfiers. Because of his work schedule, he just couldn't be "bothered" with preparing and carrying around the satisfiers. Instead, this patient used five tablets to replace a single satisfier. At only forty calories, this substitution resulted in greatly increased weight losses.

If he felt the need for additional food, he would suck on another tablet. During the twenty-one days that he followed the Super 500 program, this patient lost twelve pounds more than was considered the maximum for him.

Because he was excessively overweight, he would have had to go back on the program for an additional twenty-one-day period. Instead, this extra loss of 12 pounds resulted in his attaining his ideal weight in only an additional nine days on the program.

If you feel that you would like to use the Energizer tablets to replace the satisfiers, go ahead. The only thing to remember is to have a sufficient supply of these sweet treats available. A hundred tablets will not be sufficient. I suggest that, if you can tell how often you will be using these Energizers in your daily routine, purchase two bottles at the beginning of your program. This way you won't run into the problem of not having enough. Remember, "Be prepared."

As you can see, there are any number of ways you can substitute the Super 500 Energizer tablets for other foods. You might consider replacing a full meal with several tablets, you might substitute a satisfier with five or more of these sweet-tasting treats, or you might just use them to increase your energy level and decrease your craving for "forbidden" foods. Any way you use these tablets to achieve your ultimate goal of slenderness will be fine.

Use your imagination; incorporate these sugary-sweet tidbits into your daily routine and find out how much easier and quicker you will reach your goals.

By the way, use of the Energizers, even after you've become slender, will assist you in maintaining your new attractive physique.

CHAPTER 16

HELPFUL HINTS FOR HOLDING YOUR OWN

Most diet books attempt to illustrate how to lose excess weight without giving the least amount of thought to the problems which often arise after you've attained your goal.

It is just as important to follow a regimen *after* you've achieved slenderness as it is to do so when you are attempting to lose pounds. If you ignore the facts contained in this chapter, you will most likely begin to regain all those excess pounds you have just lost.

I know that you want to remain slender for the rest of your life, so I urge you to not disregard the information that follows.

How to Handle Those Problem Areas

Almost every patient I have ever seen has an area of their body they are not completely happy with. This may be the thighs, the stomach, the upper arms, or just about any other anatomical area. If you find yourself displeased with a specific feature of your appearance, you should take the steps necessary to correct it. Don't ever feel that you must live with some aspect of your body which displeases you.

I admit that there are certain conditions that cannot be corrected by proper nutrition or even exercise. These, however, can usually be altered sufficiently so as to pose no problem for you. If you are a woman concerned with some physical feature that dieting or exercise cannot help, I suggest you obtain one or more of the excellent beauty books that are currently on the market.

If you are a man, there is no need to feel dissatisfied with a certain feature of your appearance. Although there aren't any real "beauty" books (per se) for men, you will find adequate assistance at one of the numerous hair styling salons, men's clothiers, or health spas.

Don't become resigned to the "fact" that you have specific features with which you are unhappy. Although this book is primarily concerned with weight loss, I feel it is essential that I also offer you some advice on how to alter your appearance. I am not concerned with make-up, clothes, grace, or charm. These are areas I must leave for others to attend to. But I am interested in specific body areas that displease you.

The Importance of Anatomical Variation

Before attempting to make major changes in your appearance, you should adequately analyze your anatomy. There is nothing that will lengthen short legs or reduce the size of an over-long torso. A rib cage that is narrow or slender cannot be adequately altered to produce a massive chest. These anatomical features must be lived with.

Don't get me wrong, however. Something can be done to offset the displeasing appearance of almost any physical feature. Make-up, good grooming, and proper attire will go a long way in disguising some of the faulty features you may have.

What I am concerned with, though, are those physical traits that can be corrected. Flabby thighs, a protruding abdomen, and double chins can be altered. There is no reason for you to live with these unattractive features if you don't want to.

As I said earlier, you should, before attempting any alterations in your appearance, perform an anatomical analysis. You do this by observing your nude body in a full-length mirror. If you have been brought up in a manner that precludes your doing this, you might perform the analysis while still partially clothed, although this doesn't permit you to make a full and complete evaluation.

As you stand there observing your body, note those areas with which you are displeased. Start your analysis by looking at your feet and then allowing your eyes to proceed upward. Take into consideration each and every area. Disregard those characteristics which can't be altered through proper nutrition or exercise, and pay specific attention to those features which can be corrected.

As I mentioned previously, the anatomical variations that exist in all humans make it unlikely that any one of us will consider ourselves "perfect." For those features which cannot be changed, seek professional help in disguising them. With those features which can be sufficiently altered through proper nutrition and exercise, make a list. You will shortly learn how to correct these displeasing characteristics.

How to Bring Kinesiology to the Rescue

Kinesiology is a long word that simply means the study of movement. For instance, kinesiologists are concerned with how humans walk, what muscles come into play, and how we make various movements.

The balance of the body is extremely important when considering the kinesiological aspects of the activities we perform. You may or may not be aware that each and every movement the body is capable of has already been analyzed. Every movement you make has been categorized and studied. There are dozens of ways to perform the same act, but kinesiological studies have revealed that there is only one way that is mechanically efficient.

If you were to watch some of your acquaintances walking about and really studied how they moved, you would be surprised at how differently each one of them gets from one place to another. You may notice that one individual walks on his toes, while another walks flat-footed. You may note that the way each individual swings his or her arms while walking also differs. Some persons exaggerate the movement of their arms, while others hold them tightly by their sides.

I am sure you have noticed how some people "slink" while others "swing." Some individuals walk with their heads thrust forward, and still others walk with their heads held rigidly above their shoulders.

All of these variations in the kinesiological aspects of human motion are important. Not only do they reflect the inner emotional content of the individual (walking in a slumped position, with the head drooped on the chest, is an adequate indication that the person is not "up"), but they also reflect the amount of muscle tension that is being experienced.

If you walk properly, much of the force of gravity is overcome by the perfect balancing of the anatomical portions of the body. Much of the stress and strain of the erect posture can be absorbed by the skeletal framework of the body. Usually, however, this stress is overcome by the active participation of the muscle groups.

If you have performed your anatomical analysis correctly, you have already determined which muscle groups you are using adequately, and which muscles are not being activated.

A protruding stomach should immediately indicate that the muscles of the abdomen are not being adequately used or strengthened. Flabby thighs reveal that you are not walking as much as you should, or at least that you are walking improperly and not using all the muscle groups that should be involved.

As you proceed down the list you have formulated, you will discover any number of variants with which you are unhappy. No matter which areas are involved, an understanding of kinesiology will be helpful. Each area of the body is controlled by muscles which are responsible for the way you perform specific acts.

Take a few moments now to decide on a particular area which displeases you. Then produce some motion or movement in that area. For instance, assuming that you are dissatisfied with the size of your abdomen, you need only bend forward or back to produce some movement in this area. If you are unsure of whether you are doing this correctly, simply place one hand on the area you are attempting to activate. Once you perform the motion properly, you will actually be able to feel the contraction of the muscles under your hand, which rests on the involved area.

If you will perform this little test with each anatomical area that concerns you, you will quickly understand the kind of movements that must be made to activate each area. Once you have accomplished this, you need only repeat the actions several times until you become distinctly aware of what is required to mobilize the areas. You will then be able to do so at will.

This is basically all that is necessary to correct any physical feature with which you are unhappy. By repetitively activating those muscles which control the area involved, you will, in short order, increase the tone of both skin and muscles. You will gradually effect an alteration in the size and consistency of the anatomical feature under consideration.

Allow me to give you a few pointers about using kinesiology to affect your anatomical appearance. Assume, for the moment, that you are concerned with a protruding abdomen. If you have tried to mobilize the muscles in this area, you have become aware of what it feels like to contract the abdominal muscles. Each day, as you go about your daily activities, you can easily, voluntarily activate these muscles. Tighten up your abdomen and breathe deeply, using your chest and diaphragm. Don't allow yourself to breathe with your stomach (allowing your abdomen to rise and fall with each breath). Hold your abdomen rigid and tight, and allow your chest to expand with each respiration. You need only do this for a few minutes each day. The more often you do it, though, the quicker it will become part of your normal habits. In no time, you will unconsciously be flexing and mobilizing your abdominal muscles without being aware of it. The muscles will strengthen, the abdomen will recede, and the anatomical feature with which you were unhappy will disappear.

This method of correcting the anatomical features of your body works equally well with all muscle groups. If you are concerned about large jowls, clencing your teeth intermittently will alleviate the problem. Double chins can be easily tightened by repeatedly tensing the muscles of your neck. The same holds true for every area of your body. Just repeat the motions that activate the involved musculature, and you will soon find that you have corrected the problem areas that were bothering you.

Using the Three-Minute Total Body Revitalizer

In addition to correcting those physical characteristics you are unhappy with, you should also take part in a daily activity which strengthens and tones the entire body. I am not talking about some strenuous and boring exercise program; I am talking about a simple, pleasant procedure that takes as little as three minutes to perform.

If you have ever noticed a cat that has just awakened from sleep, you have probably been amused by the stretching movements it goes through. In essence, the cat is revitalizing its body. It is mobilizing the articulations of its skeleton, stretching the ligaments and tendons, and flexing the various muscles of its torso. Humans rarely take as much care of themselves as cats do, yet this procedure of mobilizing the entire body before starting the day is a superb method of toning up and revitalizing the body.

If you will take three minutes daily to care for your body, you will benefit from increased flexibility and circulation, you will increase the tone of your muscles, and will prepare the joints of your body for the little shocks and jolts that occur during the day.

Although I could recommend a complex and difficult procedure to follow, I have found that by simply mimicking the cat, you will more than adequately move all the joints of your body. When you awaken in the morning, prior to getting out of bed, simply turn onto your stomach and push yourself up into a kneeling position. Keeping your spine straight and level, stretch backwards until your buttocks are resting on the calves of your legs. Next, move forward until your head is in front of your arms and you feel as if you are going to fall over head first.

While in this position, stretch out one leg behind you, as if trying to touch the wall opposite your bed. Do this with the other leg. Then, get into your original position and repeat slowly. Do this several times, always attempting to get additional stretch into your movements.

When you have done this for a minute or two, stand up beside the bed. Slowly allow yourself to assume a squat posture and rest on your haunches. Flex your ankles and balance yourself on your toes. Next, raise yourself to the upright position without holding on to anything. Bring your hands above your head and stretch as much as you can, as if trying to touch the ceiling. Repeat this several times.

That's all there is to it. You needn't become an athlete to obtain benefits from some very simple movements. If you will perform these movements each morning, you will find that, throughout the day, you will feel more limber and be able to move freely.

For the two to three minutes it will take you each morning, you won't find a better "total-body revitalizer."

EPILOGUE

Although the previous chapter concludes the actual dieting information, some additional information will be of help.

In my first book on dieting, I concluded the text with a postscript or short paragraph about one of my many patients. When I inserted that material, I was unaware of the affect it would eventually have, and had no idea that so many people would identify with the young lady in that story. I hope you too will experience the changes that occurred in her life, or at least changes that are as significant.

That postscript remains to me an important reminder of the results that can be achieved by the simple expedient of losing excess weight.

It apparently also had a great effect on many of the readers who bought that first book, since I have received numerous letters, phone calls, and face-to-face compliments regarding that little episode.

Because of this, I am including another postscript at the end of this book. I think you will find it both significant and interesting, especially when you begin your own Super 500 program. I certainly hope so.

Although it was very difficult for me to choose a single patient from the great number who have benefited from the loss of weight, this particular young lady, and the problems she overcame, stand out in my mind as an example for all.

THE REBIRTH OF CANDI

When I first met Candi she was just 17 years of age. Her height, at 5'1", as well as her bone structure, which was delicate, indicated that underneath the 153 pounds she was carrying, there was a petite young girl.

Candi's parents had been patients of mine for several years, and because of this they sought my advice.

It seems that Candi, in her fifteenth year of life, had become pregnant. The religious beliefs of her family were such that she was removed from her high school and sent to an unwed mother's home.

After giving birth to a baby boy and putting him up for adoption, Candi had returned home, but her life would never be the same.

* * *

From all accounts, Candi, at age 15, had been beautiful. Although I hadn't met her at that time, I have since learned that she was considered extremely attractive. Perhaps her beauty, at least in part, was responsible for the utter degradation and self-loathing she felt. That aspect of Candi's life however, must remain untold.

The first time I saw Candi, her hair was unkempt, her clothes were in disarray, and her obesity made her look years older than she actually was. Her hair appeared dull and coarse, her skin greasy. Her finger nails had been bitten down to the quick. Candi was in need of a complete overhaul.

Her parents had brought her to me because they had been unsuccessful in helping her overcome the depression which had set in after her return home.

Candi refused to go out or to see other boys and girls her own age. She sat in her room from morning until night, gorging herself and reading.

For almost a full year prior to seeing me, she hadn't left the house, and during the previous four months, Candi had shrunken into her shell even further.

* * *

At the time of our first meeting, Candi was uncommunicative. She had even stopped speaking to her mother and father.

Her parents were frantic! They had consulted other doctors, but the recommendation that Candi be hospitalized was more than they could endure.

During the first three weeks of consultation, Candi didn't utter a word. It took more than five months of therapy before she and I could even carry on a basic conversation. After eleven months of intense therapy, Candi was once again speaking. Unfortunately, however, her depression continued, and her weight had not decreased by even a pound.

It was almost thirteen months to the day when I finally broached the subject of her obesity. Candi's response to psychological counseling had been adequate, but her obsession and depressive reaction had continued to linger. It was time to take additional steps in her behalf.

I felt that a major alteration in her appearance might be of some help. However, the reaction which I had expected when I brought up the subject of her weight didn't come. Candi seemed unconcerned with the way she looked, and I had to spend an additional forty-five minutes with her before she would even talk about trying to lose weight.

Because of her emotional and psychological state, I felt it was best not to force her into losing weight. It was something she would have to do for herself.

On the next three visits to the office, the subject of her obesity wasn't even mentioned. On the fourth visit, however, Candi brought the subject up. She had decided to take action, and wanted to lose all her fat.

Two months later, Candi weighed in at 104 pounds. Even if you could have seen the dramatic changes that took place over those eight weeks, you would still have a hard time believing it.

It wasn't only the weight loss that was dramatic: Candi's personality also changed. With every few pounds she lost, Candi became more congenial.

By the end of the first week on the Super 500 program, Candi's face was no longer bloated and puffy. Certainly it wasn't the slender, high cheek-boned face it would become over the next several weeks, but the excessive puffiness was gone. Her flesh was smooth and taut.

By the third week, Candi had dropped nineteen pounds, and her mother enticed her to go to the beauty parlor. The change was astounding! Her hair, the same hair that had appeared coarse and dry, was now glossy silk. The color hadn't been changed (it was still honey brown), but it had been cut, feathered, and styled. The effect was unbelievable. Candi looked angelic.

As the days continued to pass, Candi's weight diminished. She began wearing make-up again; not too much, but so perfectly applied, you would have to look twice to be sure she didn't have a natural blush on her cheeks. Every time she returned to my office, additional pounds had been discarded. By the end of the first month on the program, Candi was a new person.

She smiled at every turn and laughed spontaneously. There was a bounce to her walk, and the energy she radiated could actually be felt when she entered a room.

Candi bought new clothes: her taste was impeccable. Every time I saw her, I was stunned by her beauty. By the time she reached her weight goal, she could (and would) engage in conversation with just about anyone. She was no longer self-conscious. The burden of her one mistake was no longer so heavy that she could not shoulder its weight. Although Candi will probably never completely overcome her hurt or the shame she feels, she will be able to function and enjoy life.

* * *

Candi is nineteen years old now, and her life is as close to being perfect as it can be. You see, something else was taking place during the time Candi was losing weight: something that makes her story so memorable.

Unknown to Candi, her older sister, who was already married with two children of her own, had obtained custody of Candi's baby boy.

* * *

I received a letter not too long ago from Candi. She lives in Georgia now, and she has her son with her. She tells me that she's engaged to a "wonderful dude," and they plan to be married in just two months.

I know that not all the miseries and pain that afflict us can be resolved as wonderfully as Candi's. Not everyone has a sister who loves us so deeply that she would care for our child and then subsequently return him. And no, not many of us are lucky enough to find "wonderful dudes" who don't mind taking on ready-made families.

The most positive thing I can say, and perhaps the only thing that is really important, is that until Candi had worked out her emotional problems and lost her excess weight, she could not become the truly special person she is.

In all honesty, had Candi not regained her slenderness, the rest of the story would have been just as sad as the beginning.

* * *

INDEX